Nelson Yuan-sheng Kiang

Minimal Brain Dysfunction

A DEVELOPMENTAL APPROACH

Eric Denhoff, M.D.

Director, Governor Medical Center
Providence, Rhode Island

Leo Stern, M.D.

Professor of Pediatrics
Brown University, Providence, Rhode Island

MASSON Publishing USA, Inc.
New York·Paris·Barcelona·Milan·Mexico City·Rio de Janeiro

ISBN 0-89352-038-1
Library of Congress Catalog Card Number: 78-61473

Printed in the United States of America

Preface

The notion that hyperkinetic behavior is a special variety of aberrant childhood behavior stems from the early clinical studies of Charles Bradley and his colleagues. They postulated that within a spectrum of neurological dysfunctions with varying clinical manifestations, which they called syndromes of cerebral dysfunction, there was a central core of hyperkinetic behavior. Based on retrospective clinical data they found a high relationship between perinatal stress and infancy factors and the syndrome.

Socioeconomic changes following World War II resulted in an increasing number of children who would not conform to previously established standards of child behavior. It was unclear whether this change was the result of overpermissiveness in child rearing, the change in structure of the family unit, the upward-striving drives of minority groups, or overcrowded classrooms and undertrained teachers.

Subsequently, the word got around that Dexedrine or Ritalin could change inattentive behavior into organized activity. Teachers seeking solutions asked parents to seek out medical help for the child's dilemma. Physicians learned that through medication a chaotic situation at home and at school became resolved promptly. This "miracle" drug opened a Pandora's box, and soon there was an overabundance of demands upon children and overprescribing of medication on flimsy bases. Medication appeared destined to replace good teaching.

As the boundaries of hyperkinesis broadened, understandably some professionals and parents questioned the concept and the validity of managing what was at least in part perceived of as a socioeducational problem through an approach utilizing pills alone. It even became difficult for experts to compare scientific data because of the various semantic interpretations of the term. Consequently and appropriately, psychologists and educators developed alternative methods to control behavior—behavior modification. Nevertheless, there is evidence to suggest that the true hyperkinetic child cannot respond appropriately to these measures unless he or she is also given psychostimulant medication.

Now, 40 or more years after the concept of hyperkinesis was established, it is appropriate to reevaluate the events of the past in order to develop newer concepts of behavior management. Thus the developmental approach, both to the development of the problem itself and to our understanding of its origins and resolution.

The material contained herein is the result of a conference entitled Minimal Brain Dysfunction, A New Look, held under the auspices of the Department of Pediatrics at Brown University on March 2 and 3, 1977.

The contributions provide an array of information, some accepted universally, some controversial—but all practical. In different ways each contributor has had a long experience with these special children. They believe that hyperkinesis is a special entity not to be confused with developmental hyperactivity or the range of emotional disorders of childhood. None defend the abuse of psychostimulant medications and each asks that greater efforts be made in the future to help clarify and correct the reasons behind the difficulties children have in coping with modern society.

Eric Denhoff, M.D.
Leo Stern, M.D.
Providence, Rhode Island

Participants

Stanley M. Aronson, M.D., Dean of Medicine, Division of Biological and Medical Sciences, Brown University, Providence, R.I. 02912

Allan Berman, Ph.D. Professor of Psychology, Department of Psychology, University of Rhode Island, Kingston, R.I. 02881

Mr. John Coggin (Parent), 23 Pickwick Road, Marblehead, Mass. 01945

Eric Denhoff, M.D., Director, Governor Medical Center, 293 Governor Street, Providence, R.I. 02906
and Clinical Professor of Pediatrics, Brown University Medical Program, Section of Reproductive and Developmental Medicine, Brown University, Providence, R.I. 02912

Steven A. Feldman, M.D., Governor Medical Center, 293 Governor Street, Providence, R.I. 02906
and Clinical Instructor of Pediatrics, Brown University Medical Program, Section of Reproductive and Developmental Medicine, Brown University, Providence, R.I. 02912

Robert Cooke, M.D., Vice-Chancellor, Center for Health Sciences, University of Wisconsin, Madison, Wisconsin

Lester Grinspoon, MD, Associate Professor of Psychiatry, Harvard University, Boston, Massachusetts
and Massachusetts Mental Health Center, 74 Fenwood Road, Boston, Mass. 02115

Hans R. Huessy, M.D., Associate Professor of Psychiatry, Department of Psychiatry, College of Medicine, University of Vermont, Burlington, Vt. 05401

Marcel Kinsbourne, M.D., Professor of Pediatrics, Hospital for Sick Children, University Avenue, Toronto, Canada

Maurice W. Laufer, M.D. (deceased), Professor of Psychiatry, Brown University Medical Program, Section of Psychiatry, Brown University, Providence, R.I. 02912
and Emma Pendleton Bradley Hospital, Veterans Memorial Parkway, Riverside, R.I. 02915

Lucile F. Newman, Ph.D., Assistant Professor of Community Health and Anthropology, Brown University Medical Program, Section of Community Health
and Brown University, Providence, R.I. 02912

Harry S. Novack, Ph.D., Professor of Special Education, Rhode Island College, Mount Pleasant Avenue, Providence, R.I. 02908

Sigmund M. Pueschel, M.D., Assistant Professor of Pediatrics, Brown University Medical Program, Section of Reproductive and Developmental Medicine, Brown University, Providence, R.I. 02912
and Child Development Center, Rhode Island Hospital, Providence, R.I. 02902

Taranath Shetty, M.D., Clinical Assistant Professor of Pediatrics, Brown University Medical Program, Section of Reproductive and Developmental Medicine, Brown University, Providence, R.I. 02912
and 285 Governor Street, Providence, R.I. 02906

Lester Soyka, M.D., Professor of Pharmacology, Chairman of the Department of Pharmacology, College of Medicine, University of Vermont, Burlington, Vt. 05401

Leo Stern, M.D., Professor of Pediatrics, Brown University Medical Program, Section of Reproductive and Developmental Medicine, Brown University, Providence, R.I. 02912

Sumner B. Twiss, Jr., Associate Professor of Religious Studies, Brown University, Providence, R.I. 02912

Gabrielle Weiss, M.D., Associate Professor of Psychiatry, McGill University, Canada
and Department of Psychiatry, The Montreal Children's Hospital, Montreal, Canada

Sumner Yaffe, M.D., Professor of Pediatrics and Pharmacology, University of Pennsylvania
and Chairman of the Department of Pediatrics, Children's Hospital of Philadelphia, Philadelphia, Pa. 19104

Contents

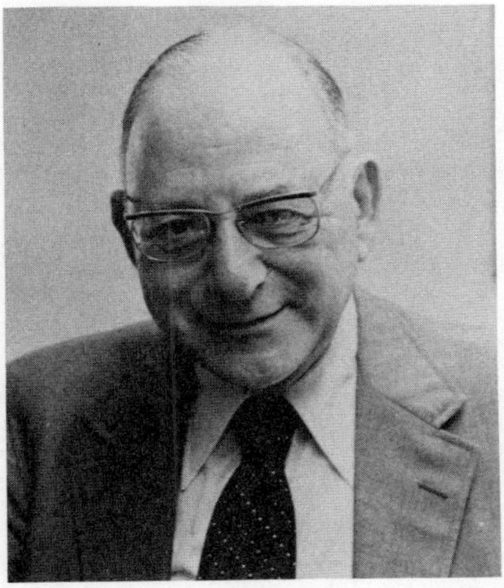

In Memoriam

We dedicate this book to Maurice W. Laufer, M.D., who recently passed away. He was a protégé of Charles Bradley and carried on the studies initiated by him. As evidenced from the chapter he wrote in this monograph, he was a superb clinician as well as a dedicated scientist.

We salute him for his many contributions to the pediatric and psychiatric literature. Most of all we will remember him for his gentleness to the large numbers of distressed children and their families. He was always there when they needed him.

Maurice W. Laufer, M.D.
May 1914—September 1978

Charles Bradley—An Appreciation

It is both fitting and proper that this symposium should be held in Providence, Rhode Island, since it was here that Charles Bradley, whom we wish to honor by this symposium, first defined the syndrome of hyperkinetic impulse disorder. With the passage of time his name and role have been associated with the Emma Pendleton Bradley Hospital, in which he worked and which today stands as an institution of renown, with much of its reputation attributable to his efforts. We wish to express our most profound appreciation.

His was an independent, significant contribution to the growth and continuance of the hospital. This has been recognized by naming one of its operating divisions and the building in which it is housed the Charles Bradley Pre-School Program located in the Charles Bradley Building. His role in the area of the hyperkinetic syndrome and its treatment requires some historical reference to the hospital and his association with it.

The institution began as the Emma Pendleton Bradley Home. Mr. and Mrs. George Lothrop Bradley desired that, because their little daughter—a beloved and only child—had suffered throughout her all-too-short life from an obscure nervous disorder, of which there was little understanding and for which there seemed to be no available treatment, other children should not suffer needlessly. As Mr. Bradley expressed it in his will; "Out of this misfortune of our only child has grown the purpose and the hope that from the affliction of this one life may come comfort and blessing to many suffering in like manner."

Following the deaths of the child and her parents, a board of trustees was organized in 1925 by the Rhode Island Hospital Trust Bank, which was both executor and trustee. Arthur H. Ruggles, M.D., was a member of this Board as well as superintendent and chief of staff, while simultaneously continuing his duties as superintendent of Butler Hospital and professor of psychiatry at Yale. On his advice, the Board agreed that the home should be for: (1) children with convulsive disorders, (2) those with behavior disorders following attacks of epidemic encephalitis, (3) those with cerebral palsy due to brain injury early in life or at birth, and (4) those with behavior disorders so severe as to necessitate isolation from the community.

An appropriate building was designed, to be situated on land which had been purchased in East Providence, and the facility was opened on April 8, 1931. From the very outset it was organized as a hospital. It was recognized that long-term care would be needed by many of the children and that the sum total of their needs had to be considered—education, recreation, family contact, etc. It was also recognized that psychotherapy would have to be a cornerstone of their treatment. This recognition, however, never led to a neglect of the importance of continuing awareness and study of the role of the central nervous system in these disorders.

In the records of the hospital Dr. Bradley, who had received pediatric as well as some psychiatric training, first appeared as Resident Physician in 1932. In 1933 he became Medical Director and in 1941 he succeeded Dr. Ruggles as Superintendent. He resigned this position in 1948 and moved to Oregon, where he still resides.

Dr. Bradley began the therapeutic use of Benzedrine, which had recently been introduced as a vasopressor, in the hope of diminishing the uncomfortable sequelae of pneumoencephalography and, being a scientist, he used it on other children as control. His scientific curiosity was aroused by some of the patients' reference to "arithmetic pills," reflecting their observation that some of them improved their performance in arithmetic while receiving this medication.

He began to investigate this phenomenon and his first paper on the topic appeared in 1937. That was exactly 40 years before the symposium which these papers celebrate, and perhaps argues against the comments of "new and untried."

In 1940 Dr. Bradley[2] wrote on school performance and psychometric performance of children receiving Benzedrine and, with Bowen, offered more general observations in 1941.[3]

In 1948, with Rosenfeld, he published his first paper delineating a behavioral syndrome with a presumably organic cause.[4] The characteristics of the syndrome were described as follows: unpredictable variability in mood, hypermotility, impulsiveness, short attention span, fluctuating ability to recall material previously learned, and conspicuous difficulty with arithmetic in school.

It was this description which stimulated us in successive attempts to define the syndrome of hyperkinetic impulse disorder and which led us to characterize a particular group of children in whom amphetamines were to prove useful.

His was the foundation upon which we built. It is to him that we would like to dedicate the proceedings of this symposium.

Eric Denhoff, M.D.
Maurice Laufer, M.D.
Providence, Rhode Island

References

1. Bradley, C.: The behavior of children receiving Benzedrine. *Am J Psychiatry* **94:** 33, 1937.
2. Bradley, C., and Green, E.: Psychometric performance of children receiving amphetamine (Benzedrine) sulfate. *Am J Psychiatry* **97:** 388–394, 1940.
3. Bradley, C., and Bowen, M.: Amphetamine therapy of children's behavior disorders. *Am J Orthopsychiatry* **11:** 92–103, 1941.
4. Rosenfeld, G.B., and Bradley, C.: Childhood behavior sequelae of asphyxia in infancy. *Pediatrics* **2:** 74–84, 1948.

MBD: A Parent's View

As the mother of a 10-year-old boy with diagnosed MBD, I have been asked to describe how this has affected our family. From birth on we suspected something was wrong with Chris. When he was diagnosed as hyperactive at the age of 4½ our suspicions were confirmed. Over the next few years he was placed on Ritalin on the basis of extensive testing. To meet his special needs in school, he was given tutorial help and sent to an elementary school out of our district. At present, he is in the regular fourth grade in the public school system, but he spends some time in a special class.

To say that Chris's condition has complicated our lives is an understatement. Trying to cope with his behavior, as well as the problems it creates, is physically, mentally, and emotionally exhausting. Generally we can say that too often it has brought us into an adversary relationship with other people, including the personnel of the school system for which we both work. Negative experiences with school personnel occur when inexperienced or overburdened teachers cannot cope with or understand our son's special needs.

In general, we seem to have a biannual battle with the department: once in the spring when we meet with an evaluation team to make out Chris's educational plan, and once in the fall when we need to make sure that it is being carried out.

In our encounters with school officials we have run into a variety of attitudes, some of which are hard to believe, coming from educators:

TEACHER:	"He can do it. He just doesn't like to."
TEACHER:	"I have to give him an incomplete. I don't know what he knows."
TEACHER:	"My students don't need to go to specialists. I can cope with them fine. I just grade them easier."
LEARNING SPECIALIST:	"Tests are a waste of time. I can see what he can do and can't do."
PRINCIPAL:	"We have no third grade teacher who can give him what he needs."
	"Well, we have nothing more to talk about." (When we would not sign Chris's educational plan)
PRINCIPAL:	"It's pushy mothers like you that cause their kids' problems."
COLLEGE PROFESSOR OF LEARNING DISABILITIES:	"The brother who's OK must have all his father's genes." (Reference to Chris's normal brother)
	"Drug therapy is dreadfully wrong."
	"Parents love to have their kids labeled LD. It's such a great excuse."

In seeking help for Chris's MBD syndrome, we have been referred to language specialists, educators, pediatricians, and psychiatrists. The inconsistencies between the various professional findings have not strengthened our confidence in the professions. Some of the attitudes and statements expressed by medical people we found confusing and unsympathetic, as the following indicate:

Pediatrician:

"They outgrow it in the same time if you try to remediate it as if you don't."

"You can try gross-motor exercises, but they don't usually change anything."

"You're at him too much. Let him do his own thing."

"You make no attempt to structure."

Pediatric Neurologist:

"He'll always be an odd duck."

"Chris's problem is essentially language."

Speech Therapist:

"We can't help him further because his problem is medical."

In the day-to-day activities that involve contact with other people, Chris's hyperactive behavior often has brought negative reactions from others as well as frustration and embarrassment to us. In stores he is apt to wander aimlessly, handle things unnecessarily and carelessly, and talk in a loud shrill voice. In other people's homes he acts in a similar manner. In restaurants his distractibility and clumsiness invariably result in spilled beverages and food. He does not know how to interact with other children, and his inappropriate behavior often brings conflicts and tears. Consequently he has few friends. Working or playing at a motor task beyond his ability brings frustration, rage, and crying fits. Adult reactions to all this include:

FRIEND: "Why not admit he is retarded."
FRIEND: "I could never stand to live with him."
FRIEND: "My professor says hyperactivity is caused by lack of love as an infant."
NEIGHBOR: "He looks normal. Are you sure there's a problem?"
RELATIVE: "You're making a mountain out of a molehill. He's not so bad."
RELATIVE: "Send him to some kind of residential school where they'll teach him how to behave."
RELATIVE: "Grin and bear it."

A family problem caused by Chris's condition is the reaction of his normal brother to our attempts to deal successfully with Chris. He is perceptive enough to realize that Chris has a problem and, at times, is capable of dealing rather sympathetically and lovingly with Chris. However, he does not understand that it is sometimes necessary to make exceptions for Chris's behavior and not for his. When we do this, he reacts with anger and resentment toward us and his brother. Consequently, to avoid this double standard, I think we tend to be somewhat permissive in our disciplinary approach toward both children. As it is, the relationship between Trip and Chris is ambivalent, involving rivalry and competition on the one hand, and brotherly love and support on the other.

Coping with all these problems is not easy. There are physical, mental, financial, and emotional strains placed upon us which are above and beyond the ordinary strains of parenthood. These include bringing Chris to a gym program for LD children twice a week, meeting the expenses of this program as well as above-average medical expenses, and planning suitable activities designed to meet his special needs. Perhaps the most exhausting strain of all is the need to carefully monitor Chris's everyday activities, including such simple tasks as getting dressed in the morning, brushing his teeth at night, or any one of a hundred things he could be doing in between. We try to do this with patience and understanding, but are not always successful.

The emotional burden of dealing with Chris's MBD is also hard to bear. At times both of us have suffered feelings of guilt, inadequacy, anger, resentment, and anxiety. We both have wondered whether one of us is responsible for Chris's condition. In particular, I have had guilt feelings regarding the time when Chris was about 6 months old. I slipped while carrying him downstairs, and he suffered a bad fall. Often I wonder if Chris's MBD could have been caused by that fall. In addition, both of us feel guilty when we lose our patience and do not deal with him calmly and lovingly. This happens more than it should.

Our failures to deal with the problems of Chris's MBD produce not only guilt, but also self-doubts concerning our roles as parents. How can we be competent parents when we cannot teach our child self-control, or when we cannot deal successfully with the problems his behavior creates? How can we be loving and caring parents when we feel angry so often? We both feel anger and resentment quite frequently. We feel angry at Chris when he fails to behave as we expect, or when he does not exhibit self-control. We feel angry at his brother when his behavior complicates matters. We feel angry at friends, neighbors, relatives, and others when they fail to understand Chris's needs. We feel angry at each other when one of us mishandles a situation or loses his patience. We feel angry toward a school system that makes us hound and demand and argue and seek for a proper educational environment for our son, an environment to which he is legally entitled but which we are made to feel unreasonable and overpowering for pursuing. And, to top it off, we feel resentment at the world for the burden of being parents of an MBD child. Why did it have to happen to us? We feel this especially when we think we see so many other parents who do not try half as hard as we do, but yet seem to have a family life with far fewer tensions.

Both of us feel anxious about Chris. We worry about him when he is not with us because we know that he can be physically hurt by others. Once a schoolmate coaxed him into putting his fingers in a desk, and then slammed the cover down on them. Chris is so trusting and eager to make friends, that he is a sitting duck for bullies. At school he is often called names, like "wierdo" or "mental." At home his brother complains that Chris's odd behavior drives away his friends. We fear for his emotional health. What can the constant negative reactions and rejections of so many people be doing to him? We would like him to grow up to be a happy person capable of functioning in, and contributing to, our society. We wonder if this will ever come to pass.

If I have sounded too negative, I do not mean to. Personally, my son has taught me to be a better teacher of high school students. I am more sensitive to their needs, more understanding of their feelings, more sympathetic about their problems, and more suited to help them achieve better education. Chris is a loving, sensitive, cooperative, and perceptive boy who tries hard to please, and who is a joy to us in so many ways. We feel he deserves a better life than he is getting.

However much we love our son, and we love him a great deal, love is not enough. It is difficult for us to live with him. It means a constant drain of our energy, time, and patience. As medical people, you can help us. We need your tolerance and understanding as friends, neighbors, and members of society.

1

Defining the Minimal Brain Dysfunction Syndrome

Maurice W. Laufer, M.D.

The term *minimal brain dysfunction* (MBD) is used to characterize the condition of children who have both specific learning disability and hyperkinetic impulse disorder.[1,2] By the former we mean impairments in learning which are not caused by inattentiveness, impairment of intelligence, sociocultural mismatch, etc., but which are due to inefficiencies in the processing of information.

Hyperkinetic impulse disorder is a behavioral picture (shortly to be described at more length) which may include school difficulties but which is due to an entirely different mechanism.

Both the specific learning disability syndrome and the hyperkinetic impulse disorder syndrome may occur together in the same child. Or one or the other may occur singly.

This flexibility in terminology may result in semantic confusion, so that one may find a learning disability sufferer being treated only with medications and a child with hyperkinetic impulse disorder being treated only by educational approaches. Such concern is supported

---

Professor of Psychiatry, Brown University Medical Program, Section of Psychiatry, Brown University, Providence; and Emma Pendleton Bradley Hospital, Riverside, Rhode Island 02915.

by a report of the use of methylphenidate in children diagnosed as having learning disability without hyperkinetic components.[2] Methylphenidate failed to improve the learning disability in these children.

What, then, is the syndrome we refer to as hyperkinetic impulse disorder?

Charles Bradley began the investigation of hyperkinesis, and his first paper on the topic appeared in November 1937: (Bradley, C.: The behavior of children receiving Benzedrine. *Am J Psychiatry* **94**:33, July 1937).

He began the use of Benzedrine, which had recently beeen introduced as a vasopressor, in the hope of diminishing uncomfortable sequelae of pneumoencephalography and, being a scientist, he used it on other children as controls. His scientific curiosity was aroused by some of the patients' reference to "arithmetic pills," reflecting their observation that some of them improved their performance in arithmetic while receiving these pills.

In 1940 he wrote on school performance and psychometric performance of children receiving Benzedrine and, with Bowen, offered more general observations in 1941.

In 1948, with Rosenfeld, he published his first paper delineating a behavioral syndrome with a presumably organic cause. (Rosenfeld, G. B., and Bradley, C.: Childhood behavior sequelae of asphyxia in infancy. *Pediatrics* 2:74-84, 1948.) The characteristics of the syndrome were described as: unpredictable variability in mood, hypermotility, impulsiveness, short attention span, fluctuant ability to recall material previously learned, and conspicuous difficulty with arithmetic in school.

It was this description which stimulated Laufer and Denhoff in their successive attempts to characterize the syndrome of hyperkinetic impulse disorder and which led them to characterize a particular group of children as those in whom amphetamines were to prove useful.

Since the manifestations of hyperkinetic may change at different ages, let us begin with a clinical description of what *might* be seen in a school age child. The word "might" should be stressed, since a given child may present all or only some of these characteristics. The estimated incidence ranges from 5 to 10 percent of school age children, and is more common in boys, especially the first born.

There may be a complaint of excessive activity. In school this may be shown by the child's inability to stay in the seat or his squirming in it, finger tapping, or roaming about the room. At home the child may be unable to sit still—even to watch television! (Though one may hear, to the contrary, that television is the only thing the child concentrates on.) Mothers often complain that the child cannot sit through a meal, dashing in for a bite and then out again. These are among the possible manifestations of *hyperactivity*.

Short attention span and poor powers of concentration are common even in the absence of hyperactivity. When observed, particularly in a group setting, this seems to be more an inability to focus attention or to inhibit distraction. All stimuli, in turn, seem equally capable of capturing attention, so that a simulus of great current importance gets no more attention than the next stimulus. Since such aspects will be diminished by an adult capturing and holding the child's attention, or by an activity of great interest chosen by the child, or at home where there is less to distract, it is often incorrectly believed that these are the signs of a spoiled child who is demanding individual attention. Instead, they are indices of distractibility.

Another frequent characteristic may be the way the child is commanded by impulse and seems unable to inhibit a response. To think of something is to do it on the spur of the moment, without reflection. A corollary is that it seems unusually difficult to delay gratification. When confronted with a test or task, the child may rush at it and through it, often not completing it. The child may dart needlessly into dangerous situations. These actions all reflect *impulsiveness.*

They may fluctuate greatly in performance, which makes for bewilderment and confusion—for them as well as for their parents, teachers, and peers. This reflects *variability* and *unpredictability*.

There may be a number of different aspects of *emotional lability*. These children may overreact emotionally, though not inappropriately, being too easily moved to laughter or to tears. They may present explosive irritability in which a small and seemingly insufficient stimulus evokes, with lightning speed, disproportionate, angry discharge from which they—but not the recipients—quickly recover.

Along with this, they may be poorly coordinated and may display difficulties in abstraction, being concrete and literal in their thinking. Their impulsiveness and distractibility may hamper their performance on tests for visual-perceptual and visual-motor capacities. Their poor and unpredictable attention may lead to spotty gaps in basic preparation. All these factors may lead to interference with learning and academic performance. This may be quite severe, but is a result of mechanisms which differ from those involved in specific learning disability *per se*.

To turn to another age group, the syndrome may also be seen in infants. Sometimes the child is recalled as having been unusually "good" and placid, possibly slow in development. More often, the infant seemed unusually sensitive to stimuli, which confront all infants, and has responded in an excessive, mass, undifferentiated way to these stimuli. As a result, the infant is querulous and irritable, cannot be soothed readily, sleeps little (day or night), and is unsatisfiable and unsatisfying—often making the mother feel frustrated and hopelessly inadequate.

These children often have a very rapid developmental schedule, getting out of the crib early and into everything. They have a great need to touch and handle objects, which often don't survive the impact. Interestingly, one of the few things that may deflect them is water—water to splash, to pour, to play in.

At the other end of the spectrum, despite persistent, erroneous statements such as "He'll grow out of it by puberty," the syndrome may definitely be present during adolescence.

By this time, the relatively clear-cut picture of earlier years may have been covered over by the effects and sequelae of many processes. Maturation may have done away with some, but not all, of the previous characteristics, while unfortunate educational and emotional sequelae persist.

The adolescent-parent problems, which are frequent in our culture, may merge with the persisting hyperkinetic remnants, covering them up, or being accentuated by them.

Studies of such adolescents frequently show poor school performance, despite adequate intelligence. The youngster often is far behind scholastically, has not been prepared properly for school, shows a great hostility to school, academic learning, and teachers, and exhibits a great deal of self-depreciation and lack of confidence.

In addition, other complaints have included the following: "Nervousness," whining, fidgetiness, poor social skills, bedwetting, preferring animals to people, refusing to obey or confirm, shunning athletics and social activities, being depressed and withdrawn, attempting suicidal, stealing, stuttering, and being assaultive and generally antagonistic.

Increasingly, despite our original assertions to the contrary, it has become obvious that this syndrome is not inevitably outgrown, but may persist into *adult* life.[3,4,5] Sometimes adults seek help because they can't concentrate on, stick to, or follow through on anything. More often, they are seen for a whole host of behaviors, distorted feelings, depression, etc. Then, on careful study, they may show impulsive behavior, restlessness, hyperactivity, concrete thinking, difficulty with mathematics or reading, liability of mood, irritability, excitability, and sometimes violent outbursts or suicidal attempts. Once recognized, the hyperkinetic components do respond favorably to Methylphenidate, amphetamines, pemoline, and imipramine.

Psychiatric Diagnosis

Diagnosis depends largely on history and reports of other observers, especially those at school. *Psychiatric interview* seeks to find evidence from observation of the presenec of hyperkinetic symptoms, to discern the possible presence of others of the syndromes of cerebral dysfunction, and to see if there is an emotional disorder present which has given rise to symptoms that mimic those of hyperkinetic impulse disorder.

Psychological testing may show a variety of subtest and scale discrepancies on the Wechsler, a discrepancy between intellectual capacity and school achievement, and impairment on the Bender Gestalt. Projective testing may reflect impulsiveness, fluidity, flow of associations, contamination, and various classical organic signs.

Differential Psychiatric Diagnosis

There has been much speculation about the possible role of depression in producing a similar symptomatic picture. Most articles on the topic of depression in children refer to a reactive neurotic rather than an endogenous psychotic depression. Those descriptions which present behavior resembling that of the hyperkinetic,[8] seem to come under the heading of "masked depression," with a question in the mind of this reader as to whether the depression might not in part be reactive to the effects of a concomitant hyperkinetic component. There is a beginning suggestion that there may be a true bipolar depression in early adolescence, with a true manic component. If so, as yet this seems to be rare.

Other possibilities which need to be differentiated include the following: the presence and effect of anxiety and inner tension, boredom in class, sociocultural mismatch, hypoglycemia, asocially and familially induced hyperaggressiveness, hyperthyroidism, secondary reaction to scholastic incapacity, and acting out of pathological family dynamics.

Conclusion

Hyperkinetic impulse disorder is a fairly common entity. Its behavioral manifestations frequently evoke emotional consequences in the child, family, and teachers. It may also be accompanied by or lead to scholastic difficulties. Because it may last for several years and its manifestations and complications may be manifold, its study and treatment call for much of the art as well as much of the science of medicine.

References

1. Denhoff, E., Laufer, M.W., and Holden, R.H.: The syndromes of cerebral dysfunction. *J Okla State Med Assoc* **52:** 360–366, 1959.
2. Gittelman-Klein, R., and Klein, D.F.: Methylphenidate effects in learning disabilities. *Arch Gen Psychiatry* **33:** 655–664, 1976.
3. Hartocollis, P.: The syndrome of minimal brain dysfunction in young adult patients. *Bull Menninger Clin* **32:** 102–114, 1968.
4. Quitkin, F., and Klein, D.F.: Two behavioral syndromes in young adults related to possible minimal brain dysfunction. *J Psychiatr Res* **7:** 131–142, 1969.
5. Mann, H.B., and Greenspan, S.I.: The identification and treatment of adult brain dysfunction. *Am J Psychiatr* **133:** 1013–1017, 1976.
6. Laufer, M.W., Denhoff, E., and Rubin, E.A.: Photo-Metrazol activation in children. *Electroencephalogr Clin Neurophysiol* **6:** 1–8, 1964.
7. Satterfield, J.H., Lesser, L.I., Saul, R.E., and Cantwell, D.P.: Electroencephalographic aspects in the diagnosis and treatment of minimal brain dysfunction. *Ann NY Acad Sci* **205:** 274–282, 1973.
8. Cytryn, L., and McKnew, D.H., Jr.: Proposed classification of childhood depression. *Am J Psychiatry* **129:** 149–155, 1972.
9. Corson, S.A., et al. Effects of D-amphetamine on hyperkinetic, untrainable dogs. *Fed Proc* **30:** 1971.
10. Corson, S.A., et al.: Experimental control of hyperkinetic and violent behavior in dogs. Black and white sound film, 16 mm, narrated by L.E. Arnold, 1972.

2

Psychopharmacology in Childhood and Adolescence

Michele Danish, Pharm.D. and Sumner J. Yaffe, M.D.*

Introduction

The classification of psychotropic or psychoactive agents for use in children and adolescents is greatly hampered by the lack of data regarding their safety and efficacy. Despite the almost explosive introduction of these agents into the marketplace over the past several decades, evaluation in the child has not proceeded concomitantly. In the past, results from psychiatric drug usage in adults had been so encouraging that it was readily accepted that one could apply the same methods of therapy to children; stimulants, anti-depressants, and tranquilizers are now being prescribed for children with various mental disorders. Although there has always been apprehension about using these drugs in children, because of the possible permanent effects the drugs may have on later behavior, growth, and intelligence, there have been very few well-controlled studies establishing the

Division of Clinical Pharmacology, Department of Pediatrics, University of Pennsylvania School of Medicine and Children's Hospital of Philadelphia, Philadelphia, Pennsylvania.

* Reprint requests to S. J. Yaffe.

safety, efficacy, dosage requirements, and disposition of this group of drugs in children.

Reasons for this gap in knowledge are manifold. Of utmost importance is the inability to diagnose and classify childhood mental illness. As a consequence, drug evaluation, even if attempted, has been carried out badly because of the nonrigorous nature of the clinical trial. Problems peculiar to drug evaluation in children, such as the ethical considerations of experimenting on minor (especially if they are mentally retarded), have contributed to the lack of scientific data on the effects of psychotropic drugs on children. Other major factors responsible for the current status of pediatric psychopharmacology include the lack of pediatric clinical pharmacologists and the unavailability of adequate analytical methods, including micro methods, stable isotopes, and noninvasive approaches, which would have facilitated drug evaluation in the minor subject.

Through repetitive use over the years, certain drugs (e.g., amitriptyline for enuresis,[43] amphetamine for MBD[11]) have been shown in placebo-controlled studies to be definitely effective in illnesses peculiar to childhood. In general, however, determination of drug effectiveness has been very subjective. Even more subjective have been the dosages prescribed for pediatric patients. Adjustment of the adult dose solely by body weight is inaccurate and has resulted in both toxicity and insufficient dosing of psychiatric drugs.[19]

At the same time, impressive advances have been made in our understanding of the action of disposition of psychotropics in adult patients: "steady-state" plasma and serum drug concentrations have been correlated in many instances with drug effects. Drug dosages have been modified to take into consideration variations in rate of metabolism and elimination, the extent of drug protein-binding interaction with other drugs, and individual variations in drug response. The sophisticated and rational use of these compounds in the adult starkly contrasts with the empiric approach employed in the management of the sick infant or child.

The distribution and elimination of the psychoactive drugs in children may play a very important role in explaining differences seen in efficacy and safety between pediatric and adult patients. This is of particular significance with the psychoactive drugs because most of these drugs are highly bound to various body tissues (brain, liver, fat) and plasma proteins and they have active metabolites.[10] Although the disposition of psychiatric drugs in children has not been studied, there have been many recent reports that drug disposition does differ with age. Antipyrine, phenylbutazone,[2] acetaminophen,[12] and theophylline[15] are eliminated more rapidly in children. Protein binding may also change with age, since diphenylhydantoin protein binding has been shown to change during adolescence.[3] In addition, children generally have less adipose tissue than adults.

Since assay methods are available for many of the psychoactive drugs, it should now be possible to answer many of these questions concerning disposition in children. The ideal method for determining the correct dosage for children would come from measurement of drug concentrations at the presumed site of activity (e.g., the central nervous system) and in the serum. This would be of great value in establishing a dose-serum level-responsive curve. Since this information is not presently available, it is still necessary to use general pediatric guidelines for dosing and for measuring safety and efficacy.

Nonetheless, it is not too optimistic to consider that pediatric psychopharmacology will change with the acquisition of a data base from careful clinical trials. The classification we have employed is predicated on this assumption, as a result of which the drugs have been characterized according to accepted use (psychoses, affective disorders, anxiety, and behavioral syndromes). Within each clinical situation further classification has been derived from chemical structure. Dosage recommendations in children have been purposefully not made since these are discussed in the individual chapters covering specific usage in childhood mental illness. When disposition and pharmacodynamic data are available in children they are mentioned in addition to side-effects and cautions which we think should be observed because of the stage of development of the child and the manner in which this may influence drug action and disposition.

Antipsychotic Agents

Three structural classes of psychotropic drugs are currently employed in the therapy of childhood and adolescent schizophrenia. These include the phenothiazines, the thioxanthenes, and the butyrophenones. Their pharmacologic properties, disposition, and side-effects are discussed in the following paragraphs.

The Phenothiazines

The phenothiazines as a class are not only among the most widely used therapeutic agents but they also appear to have the greatest array of pharmacologic effects, exerting an action on most organ systems. The phenothiazines consist of a triple-ring heterocyclic nucleus, in which two benzene rings are linked by both a sulfur and a nitrogen atom. Although many phenothiazine derivatives have been developed in the search for better antipsychotic medication, most are of equivalent potency.

The phenothiazines can be subdivided into three groups on the basis of substitution on the nitrogen atom in position 10 in the middle ring. All substituted groups contain nitrogen, either in ring or chain form. Chlorpromazine, the most widely used and hence the prototype of the phenothiazines, has an aliphatic (aminoalkyl) side chain. Thioridazine, widely used as an adjunct in the management of the hyperactivity of psychotic children, is a member of the second group with a piperidine side chain. The other subgroup is the piperazine substituted group represented by prochlorperazine (Compazine) and fluphenazine. All the phenothiazines used as antipsychotic agents have a three-carbon bridge between the nitrogen atom of the middle ring and that of the side chain. This is in contrast to the anticholinergic phenothiazines used in the management of parkinsonism and the antihistaminic phenothiazines, which have only two carbons separating the nitrogen of the middle ring from the nitrogen of the side chain or ring.

The phenothiazines have diverse effects on the central nervous system, varying from slowing of EEG patterns and increase in occurrence of theta waves to blockade of the chemoreceptor trigger zone of the medulla from the emetic effects of apomorphine, a dopamine receptor stimulant. Considerable research has generated many hypotheses concerning the precise mechanism of action of the phenothiazines. The most attractive of these theories and the one which correlates well with antipsychotic activity involves blockade of dopamine mediated synaptic transmission.[38] This mechanism may also explain how these drugs evoke parkinsonian-like extrapyramidal neurologic symptoms. Animal studies have demonstrated that phenothiazines inhibit dopamine activation of adenylate cyclase in both the caudate nucleus and the limbic system. While this may be the dopamine receptor for the drug, the precise role of dopamine in the etiology of schizophrenia has not been established.

The disposition of the phenothiazines within the organism depends on the particular drug molecule. Chlorpromazine is discussed because of its widespread usage and thorough investigation. Peak plasma concentrations are found within several hours after oral administration. Elimination is almost entirely via hepatic metabolism into a large number of different metabolites. The plasma half-life of the parent drug is less than 6 hours, but metabolites are excreted for weeks after cessation of administration. This is perhaps due to storage and distribution in lipid, especially in the brain, where much higher concentrations are achieved than in plasma. There has been considerable research attempting to correlate blood concentrations with therapeutic response.[22] The 7-hydroxy derivative may correlate best with clinical effect. These correlations are confounded not only by the large numbers of metabolites but also by the fact that psychotic patients continue to show beneficial effects long after the drugs have been discontinued. More recently, a specific sensitive gas–liquid chromatography (GLC) assay method for chlorpromazine has been developed.[45] Improvement, as determined by a psychiatric rating scale, was found only in those patients with high plasma concentrations of 150–300 ng/ml. Patients with lower concentrations had no clinical improvement, while toxicity in the form of tremors and convulsions occurred with very high levels (750–1000 ng/ml). While there are a few well-controlled studies of chlorpromazine efficacy in schizophrenic children at dosages of 2–9 mg/kg/day,[31] there are no studies of its disposition in the pediatric patient.

Since the many phenothiazine derivatives have similar clinical effects, the major differences relate to the nature and extent of side effects. Potency appears to increase from the piperidine to the aminoalkyl to the piperazine substituted drugs. Thus a continuum of side effects can be constructed with thioridazine at one end extending to chlorpromazine to perphenazine to fluphenazine. Sedation is greatest at the thioridazine end and least with fluphenazine, while neurologic effects are the opposite. These variations can be taken into consideration when patients manifest adverse effects. Granular deposits in the cornea have been seen in adult patients on very high doses of chlorpromazine. The major side effect of chronic administration is tardive dyskinesia.[35] These neurologic signs include athetoid movements of the hands, vermicular movements of the tongue, or tics of the lips or jaw. They are most often seen in older patients in whom drug metabolism may be altered. Cessation of therapy does not necessarily eliminate the adverse effects and the drugs may have to be continued, with acceptance of the neurologic effects.

The Thioxanthenes

The thioxanthenes are structural derivatives of the phenothiazines, with replacement of the nitrogen atom in the molecule at position 10 by a carbon atom. Those thioxanthenes with central nervous system activity are characterized by a double bond between the C10 and the side chain as well as by substitutions in position 2.

While many thioxanthenes have been synthesized, only two are available for clinical use in the United States: chlorprothixene, an analogue of chlorpromazine, and thiothixene, an analogue of thioproperazine. It should be noted that, because of a double bond at C10, two isomers of each substituted thioxanthene can be formed. These have been separated and the cis form is much more pharmacologically active than the trans isomer. Both thioxanthenes have actions similar to those of their phenothiazine analogues. While clinical studies of their efficacy, particularly in schizophrenic patients, abound, there are no data on disposition available. The studies of thiothixene in schizophrenic children are noteworthy because of the presence of antipsychotic activity without sedation, a major drawback with chlorpromazine therapy.[20] A dosage of 6–30 mg/day (mean, 14 mg/day) was efficacious in the management of 10 psychotic boys aged 5–15 years.[47] The improvement in behavior (emotional unresponsiveness, mood lability, attention span, motor activity, and socialization) correlated with improvement in EEG patterns. Extrapyramidal signs, one of the major adverse effects in adults, are less common in children.

The Butyrophenones

While many butyrophenones have been synthesized and evaluated since the discovery of the neuroleptic and antipsychotic actions of this class, only two compounds are currently approved for use in the United States: haloperidol and droperidol. The latter has a very short duration of action and is used only as an adjunct to general anesthesia. Although structurally different from the phenothiazines, the butyrophenones share many of their pharmacologic properties. Haloperidol is an extremely potent antipsychotic, which has been shown to be effective in the treatment of both manic illness and schizophrenia. Its mechanism of action is considered to be similar to that of the phenothiazines since it also blocks the effects of dopamine.

Haloperidol has been extensively used in child psychiatry. Two studies have compared its effectiveness in schizophrenic children with that of fluphenazine. In one investigation haloperidol in doses up to 16 mg/day was successful in reducing autism and provocative behavior.[18] In the other study there were considerably fewer extrapyramidal side effects with haloperidol than with the phenothiazines.[16]

The disposition of the drug is unknown in children. Studies in man are incomplete. The drug appears to be rapidly absorbed from the gastrointestinal tract, with peak plasma concentrations reached at 2 hours. Elimination occurs only after prior metabolism in the liver. It is important to note that no correlation was found between therapeutic response and plasma concentration of the parent drug.[52]

Side effects appear to be dose related and, on the whole, consist of extrapyramidal reactions. These were of a low incidence in the two pediatric studies cited above.

Stimulants

The pediatric clinical syndromes of hyperkinesis and minimal brain dysfunction are characterized by motor restlessness, impulsiveness, learning difficulty, and a low frustration tolerance.[14] Although not all children benefit from stimulant drug therapy and the use of stimulants in children is controversial, controlled studies have shown the efficacy of stimulants in certain children and a 4- to 8-week trial of drug therapy is often worthwhile. The stimulants most often employed are dextroamphetamine, methylphenidate, and pemoline.

Amphetamines

Amphetamines have been used for almost 40 years in the treatment of children with behavior disorders.[9] Amphetamines are sympathomimetic phenylethylamines that are powerful CNS stimulants, in addition to having peripheral alpha and beta adrenergic activity. The D isomer has greater CNS effects and less cardiovascular effects than the L isomer and is the form most often administered to children.

The mechanism of action of amphetamines in behavioral disorders has not been clearly identified. Amphetamines do act to promote the release and prevent the reuptake of monoamines from the neurons; it is probably through this effect on CNS neurotransmitters that amphetamines enhance the functioning of the reticular activating system and thereby improve the behavior reinforcement system mediated through cortical inhibition.[6,49]

Amphetamines are readily absorbed after oral administration and are rapidly distributed to tissues, especially the kidneys, lungs, and brain.[33] The half-life of amphetamine has been reported to be approximately 5 hours in adults with an acidic urine.[7] Serum half-life increases with chronic use. About 35–40% of amphetamine is excreted unchanged in an alkaline pH; acidic urine increases excretion of the unchanged drug to 70%.[4] Amphetamine is metabolized by two major pathways in man, oxidative deamination and hydroxylation. It has been suggested that the hydroxylation pathway is responsible for production of false neurotransmitters and that these metabolites are retained in the body longer than the parent drug.

There have been no studies done in hyperkinetic children to determine if there are differences in the disposition of drug from adults. However, Epstein and his co-workers[17] monitored urinary excretion of dextroamphetamine and found a higher percentage of unchanged drug in the responders as compared to nonresponders at 7 hours after administration. Further studies are needed to determine if hyperkinesis or the age of the patient effects drug metabolism.

Side effects are reported in approximately 10–15% of children taking amphetamines, but they are usually not serious enough to warrant discontinuation of therapy.[40] The most serious effect is psychosis with hallucinations. The degree of psychosis has been directly related to the concentration of the hydroxylated amphetamine metabolites in the urine.[5] Although rare, psychosis has been reported in children.[42] Anorexia and weight loss are common at doses greater than 15 mg/day,[19] but tolerance to these effects and to the insomnia usually develops within 1 to 2 weeks. Chronic administration may suppress growth and this should be carefully monitored.

Dizziness, irritability, cardiac arrhythmias, and nausea and vomiting have been observed after accidental ingestion.

Long-term safety in children has not been ascertained. This is of particular importance with drugs that effect the CNS and are used for months to years during a period of continuous brain development and maturation.

Methylphenidate

Methylphenidate is a piperidine derivative of amphetamine. The pharmacologic and behavioral properties are essentially the same as those of amphetamine.[36] Methylphenidate is at least equally effective[11] and possibly more effective[40] than dextroamphetamine in the treatment of hyperkinetic children.

The metabolic fate of methylphenidate in man has not yet been elucidated, however methylphenidate may influence the metabolism of other drugs, including the anticonvulsants.[23]

Side effects are seen in about 14 percent of children treated with methylphenidate.[40] This is similar to the amount of side effects seen with dextroamphetamine, however there is probably less suppression of weight gain with methylphenidate.[46] Acute episodes of psychosis and hallucinations have also been reported with methylphenidate.[32]

Pemoline

Magnesium pemoline is an oxazolidine derivative which has been introduced into pediatrics as an alternative to the amphetamine-like drugs for the treatment of hyperkinesis. Its chemical structure differs from that of amphetamine and methylphenidate and it has no sympathomimetic activity.

Pemoline is a CNS stimulant and, although its mechanism of action in man is not known, it does increase dopamine synthesis in the rat brain.

The half-life of pemoline averages 12 hours and once-a-day dosing is usually sufficient. In two placebo-controlled studies,[11] pemoline was effective in treating MBD, with the maximum response observed after 6 weeks of therapy.

The reported side effects have been most often related to the drug's CNS stimulatory effects: anorexia, insomnia, restlessness, dizziness, and headaches. Initial weight loss has been reported to return to the normal weight gain curve after 3–6 months of drug administration. Psychosis has been reported in adults after chronic administration. There have been no long-term studies of pemoline's effect on growth and, until such data become available, the growth rate should be monitored in all patients.

Antidepressants

The Tricyclic Antidepressants

The tricyclic antidepressants, represented by imipramine, amitryptyline, and their demethylated metabolites, desipramine and nortriptyline, are used in the treatment of children with depression, hyperactive-agressive behavior, or enuresis.

The mechanism of action in the management of any of these conditions has not been ascertained. However, it is known that the tricyclics inhibit the neuronal uptake of monoamines. It has been theorized that depression may be caused by insufficient quantities of norepinephrine or serotonin at CNS receptor sites and, by preventing the reuptake of norepinephrine and serotonin by the nerve terminal, more of these amines are available at the presumed site of activity. Although it is known that the demethylated tricyclics are more potent in the blockade of norepinephrine and the methylated drugs are more effective in the blockade of serotonin reuptake, the clinical significance of this differential is not clear. It has also been demonstrated that in animals higher doses of tricyclics may actually antagonize the effects of norepinephrine on the adrenergic receptors,[27] which may in part account for the side effects seen with the tricyclics at higher doses.[48]

The mechanism by which the tricyclics act in enuresis is even less well understood. It has been postulated that in addition to their effect on mood, their anticholinergic and central stimulant properties may play a role in alleviating enuresis.[43]

The tricyclics are rapidly and completely absorbed after oral administration. However, only 29–77% of imipramine[24] and 46–60% of nortriptyline[25] are systematically available because the drugs are metabolized in the liver before entering the general systemic circulation (first pass effect).

It requires 2–3 weeks of daily administration to see a therapeutic response to the tricyclics. This corresponds to the duration of time needed to reach steady-state plasma levels because of long half-lives (imipramine half-lives in children range from 25 to 60 hours).[51]

Steady-state plasma levels show large variations in patients on equivalent doses.[48] This can be attributed to variance in the rate of metabolism and, to a lesser extent, to differences in protein binding. The rate of metabolism is genetically determined and may also be affected by exposure to other drugs.[1]

It is the amount of free drug which is considered the active component available at the site of action. Therefore, the protein binding of imipramine, which changes with age, may be very important in determining dosage requirements: 26% is free in the neonate, 14 to 22% in the 7- to 10-year-old group and 5–23% free in depressed adult patients.[51]

The tricyclics are fat soluble and have a large volume of distribution (about 15–30 l./kg in the adult).[48] Children generally have smaller adipose compartments than adults, however, and this may increase the amount of drug available to the CNS.[51]

In adults, the tricyclics have an overall adverse reaction rate of 15%, while major adverse reactions (psychosis, hallucinations, etc.) occur in 4.6%.[8] The most commonly reported complaints are related to the anticholinergic effects of the drugs and include dry mouth, decreased gut motility, and urinary retention.

In addition to the anticholinergic effects, the tricyclics have an affinity for cardiac tissue and may cause direct myocardial depression. Other cardiovascular findings include decreased cardiac output and increased duration of the QRS complex on electrocardiograms.[50]

In summary, the tricyclic antidepressants are useful drugs in children, especially for the treatment of enuresis. The disposition studies done in children illustrate the importance of determining dose–response relationships in this age group and the error that can occur from extrapolation from adult data. Since the safety and efficacy of various suggested dosage regimens for children have not been thoroughly studied, children should be carefully monitored while receiving medication, particularly with long-term administration. Doses of 1–2 mg/kg/day have been established for enuresis. While higher doses have been used as an antidepressant, doses above this level may be unsafe and patients should be carefully monitored for electrocardiographic abnormalities.

The Monoamine Oxidase (MAO) Inhibitors

The MAO inhibitors, which include the hydrazide derivatives (isocarboxacid, nialamide, and phenelzine) and the nonhydrazides (tranylcypromine and pargyline), have been used in the past for the treatment of depression and narcolepsy. Because of the high potential for toxicity and the disputed efficacy of this group of drugs, their use in recent years has greatly diminished. However, the MAO inhibitors do offer an alternative method of therapy for patients with atypical endogenous depression which does not respond to the drugs of choice, i.e., the tricyclics.[29]

The MAO enzymes are located primarily within the neuron and are major regulators of epinephrine, norepinephrine, dopamine, and serotonin metabolism. The MAO inhibitors irreversibly inactivate the isoenzymes that deaminate the monoamines and allow an increase in intracellular amine levels. The correlation of their pyschological effects with this physiologic effect has not yet been demonstrated, despite considerable research. The MAO inhibitors, particularly phenelzine and tranylcypromine, have been reported to elevate the mood of depressed patients and to suppress REM sleep. As with the tricyclics, it takes several weeks of daily administration for a response to be observed; this is probably because their activity depends on the rate of enzyme synthesis. Prospective studies are still needed to evaluate their role in pediatric psychiatry.

The MAO inhibitors are lipophilic compounds which are absorbed from the gut and readily cross the blood–brain barrier. The hydrazide derivatives are thought to be cleaved before activation. Phenelzine is probably dehydrazinated to phenylacetic acid by an MAO catalyzed reaction.[28] The nonhydrazine group combines directly with the MAO isoenzymes and, unlike with the hydrazide group, this union may be slowly reversible. The hydrazide group is deactivated by acetylation; about half the adult population are slow acetylators of phenelzine, which may effect the observed response to the drug.[30]

The toxicity reported with the MAO inhibitors has been the major factor responsible for decreased use of these drugs. Although all the drugs in this group can potentially cause severe adverse reactions, the two drugs now in common use, phenelzine and tranylcypromine, rarely cause any serious problems.[44]

With an acute overdose, symptoms occur in a few hours and are usually characterized by agitation, hallucinations, hyperpyrexia, convulsions, and occasionally coma and death. Both increases and decreases in blood pressure are observed. Dialysis may be of value in decreasing the serum levels.[37]

Hepatotoxicity, which is not dose related, has been reported in patients on chronic therapy. Other side effects reported with long-term therapy include tremors, insomnia, peripheral neuropathy, and orthostatic hypotension.[10] Less serious complaints have included headaches, dizziness, fatigue, constipation, and urinary retention.

The various cardiovascular and autonomic side effects observed with MAO inhibitor administration are usually tolerable; however, a greater possibility for toxicity occurs in their interaction with food and other drugs. MAO inhibitors potentiate the effect of peripherally acting amines, particularly amphetamines and tyramine. It is of the utmost importance to alert patients to this interaction because a hypertensive crisis may occur if the patient ingests foods containing tyramine (cheeses, beer, wines, liver, pickled herring, tripe, yeast, coffee, canned figs, or large portions of any dairy product).[34]

MAO inhibitors also inhibit liver enzymes other than MAO and therefore could inhibit the metabolism of anesthetics, barbiturates, and narcotics.[13]

In summary, the administration of MAO inhibitors to children should be approached with extreme caution because of the lack of data in children and the reported adverse reactions in adults.

Tranquilizers

A number of different classes of pharmacologic agents are used in children with anxiety and neurotic symptoms. The drugs most frequently prescribed are the benzodiazepines (diazepam, chlordiazepoxide, clorazepate, flurazepam, and oxazepam) and the antihistamine sedatives (hydroxyzine and diphenhydramine). The propanediol carbamates, meprobamate and tybamate, are used so rarely (and for other indications) as not to warrant discussion.

The benzodiazepines have been the subject of a recent review.[26]

They are very widely used, but no breakdown is available concerning age distribution of usage. Thirty percent of medical inpatients in two Boston teaching hospitals monitored by the Boston Collaborative Drug Surveillance Program in 1973 received diazepam and 32% flurazepam. Outpatient usage is just as frequent, with 77 million prescriptions filled in retail pharmacies in 1972.

The various benzodiazepine derivatives have qualitatively similar properties despite variations in potency. The behavioral effects seen in animals following benzodiazepine administration have been collectively termed *disinhibition.* These include an increase in spontaneous and exploratory activity, reduction of the suppressive effects of punishment, and attenuation of the behavioral sequelae of stress. These are mentioned because clinical antianxiety effects of drugs are speculated to be the counterpart of disinhibition in animals. These procedures are used for screening and development of new compounds. It is noteworthy that behavioral effects in animals produced by the benzodiazepines occur at low dosages whereas nonspecific central nervous system depression requires much larger dosages. Although meprobamate and barbiturates also produce disinhibition they do so at very close to toxic doses. The antipsychotic agents (see above) do not produce disinhibition in animals at any dose.

Diazepam is rapidly absorbed following oral administration, with a peak level occurring at 2 hours. The intramuscular route should not be used because of very erratic absorption. The drug is slowly metabolized to the desmethyl derivative (half-life, 1–2 days). This active compound is subsequently hydroxylated (oxazepam) and rapidly glucuronidated before renal excretion. Steady-state concentrations are reached about a week after initiation of therapy. Diazepam disposition in children is somewhat more rapid than in adults with a plasma half-life of 18 hours.[41] Because of the relatively slow rates of metabolism, diazepam and chlordiazepoxide can be given one to two times/day. Oxazepam, with a rapid biotransformation to inactive metabolites, requires three to four doses/day. The slowly metabolized compounds tend to accumulate with clinical effects or toxicity not apparent until 7–10 days after the initiation of therapy. Similarly, effects may be evident for some time after the cessation of therapy. These pharmacokinetic properties must be kept in mind when dosages are altered. Toxic reactions and side effects are minimal with these compounds. This is undoubtedly a major reason for their widespread usage. Drowsiness, the most common side effect, is an extension of the pharmacologic action and can be eliminated by reduction of dosage.

The antihistamine sedatives continue to be used in pediatric practice. Diphenhydramine is effective in young children as an antianxiety agent, irrespective of the presence of hyperactivity.[21] At puberty, effectiveness decreases and an increased dose is associated with drowsiness. For this reason, it is used as a bedtime sedative in this age group. The effectiveness of hydroxyzine in the management of anxiety is less clear. There are conflicting reports as to whether or not it is better than a placebo in adult subjects. There are, however, no studies reported in children, and usage in this age group cannot be recommended.[39]

References

1. Alexanderson, B., Sjoqvist, F., and Price Evans, D.: Steady state plasma levels of nortriptyline in twins: Influence of genetic factors and drug therapy. *Br Med J* **4:** 764, 1969.
2. Alvares, A.P., Kapelner, S., Sassa, S., and Kappas, A.: Drug metabolism in normal children, lead-poisoned children, and normal adults. *Clin Pharmacol Ther* **17:** 179, 1975.
3. Andritz, M., and Jusko, W.: Personal communication (1975).
4. Anggard, E., Gunne, L., Jonsson, L., and Niklasson, F.: Pharmacokinetic and clinical studies on amphetamine dependent subjects. *Eur J Clin Pharmacol* **3:** 3, 1970.
5. Anggard, E., Jonsson, L., Hogmark, A., and Gunne, L.: Amphetamine metabolism in amphetamine psychosis. *Clin Pharmacol Ther* **14:** 870, 1973.
6. Baldessarani, R.J.: Pharmacology of the amphetamines. *Pediatrics* **49:** 694, 1972.
7. Beckett, A.H.: Drug metabolism and kinetics of sympathomimetic amines in man. In *The Present Status of Psychotropic Drugs*, A. Cerletti and F. Bove, Eds. Excerpta Medica Foundation, 1969.
8. Boston Collaborative Drug Surveillance Program: Adverse reactions to the tricyclics antidepressant drugs. *Lancet* **1:** 529, 1972.
9. Bradley, C.: The behavior of children receiving Benzedrine. *Am J Psychiatry*, **94:** 577, 1937.
10. Byck, R.: Drugs and the treatment of psychiatric disorders. In *The Pharmacological Basis of Therapeutics* (5th ed.). L.S. Goodman and A. Gilman, Eds. Macmillan, New York, 1975.
11. Conners, C.K.: Recent drug studies with hyperkinetic children. *J Learn Disabil* **4:** 476, 1971.
12. Danish, M., and Yaffe, S.: Acetaminophen disposition in adolescents [abstract]. *Pediatr Res* **9:** 283, 1975.
13. Eade, N.R., and Renton, K.W.: The effect of phenelzine and tranylcypromine on the degradation of meperidine. *J Pharmacol Exp Ther* **173:** 31–36, 1970.
14. Eisenberg, L.: The clinical use of stimulant drugs in children. *Pediatrics* **49:** 709, 1972.
15. Ellis, E.F., Levy, G., and Koysooko, R.: Pharmacokinetics of theophylline in children. (Submitted for publication.)
16. Engelhardt, D.M., Polizoes, P., Waizer, J., and Hoffman, S.P.: A double-blind comparison of fluphenazine and haloperidol in out-patient schizophrenic children. *J Autism Child Schizo* **3:** 128–127, 1973.
17. Epstein, L.C., Lasagna, L., and Conners, C.K.: Correlation of dextroamphetamine excretion and drug response in hyperkinetic children. *J Nerv Ment Dis* **146:** 136, 1968.
18. Faretra, G., Droher, C., and Dowling, J.: Comparison of haloperidol and fluphenazine in disturbed children. *Am J Psychiatry* **126:** 146–149, 1970.
19. Fish, B.: Drug therapy in children's psychiatric disorders. *Mod Prob Pharmacopsychiatry* **1:** 60, 1968.
20. Fish, B., Campbell, M., Shapiro, T., and Weinstein, J.: Preliminary find-

ings on thiothixene compared to other drugs in psychotic children. *Moddern Problems of Pharmacopsychiatry*. H.E. Lehmann and T.A. Ban Karger, Eds. Basel, 1969.
21. Fish, B., and Shapiro, T.: A typology of children's psychiatric disorders: Its application to a controlled evaluation of treatment. *J Am Acad Child Psychiatry* **4:** 32–52, 1965.
22. Forrest, I.S., Carr, C.J., and Usdin, E.: *Phenothiazines and Structurally Related Drugs*. Raven Press, New York, 1974.
23. Garretson, L.K., Perel, J.M., and Dayton, P.G.: Methylphenidate interaction with both anticonvulsants and ethylbiscoumacetate. *JAMA* **207:** 2052, 1969.
24. Gram, L., and Christiansen, J.: First pass metabolism of imipramine in man. *Clin Pharmacol Ther* **17:** 555, 1975.
25. Gram, L., and Overo, K.: First pass metabolism of nortriptyline in man. *Clin Pharmcol Ther* **18:** 305, 1975.
26. Greenblatt, D.J., and Shader, R.I.: Benzodiazepines. *N Eng J Med* **291:** 1011–1015, 1974.
27. Haefly, W., Hurlimann, A., and Thoesen, H.: Scheenbar paradoxe beeinflussung von peripheren noradrenaliniverkungen durch einige thymoleptika. *Helv Physiol Acta* **22:** 15, 1964.
28. Horita, A., Clineschmidt, B.V., and McMonigle, J.J.: The role of metabolism in the action of some monoamine oxidase inhibitors In *The Present Status of Psychotropic Drugs*, A. Cerletti and F.J. Bove, Eds. Excerpta Medica Foundation, Amsterdam, 1969.
29. Johnson, W. C.: *Dis Nerv Sys* **36:** 521, 1975.
30. Johnston, E.C., and Marsh, W.: Acetylator status and response to phenelzine in depressed patients. *Lancet* **1:** 567, 1973.
31. Kurem, J., Fish, B., Shapiro, T., Gerner, E.W., and Levidow, C.: EEG and behavioral effects on drug therapy in children: Chlorpromazine and diphenhydramine. *Arch Gen Psychiatry* **24:** 552, 1971.
32. Lucas, A.R., and Weiss, M.: Methylphenidate hallucinosis. *JAMA* **217:** 1079, 1971.
33. Maikel, R.P., Cox, R.H., Miller, F.P., Segal, D.S., and Russell, R.W.: Correlation of brain levels of drugs with behavioral effects. *J Pharmacol Exp Ther* **165:** 216, 1969.
34. Marley, E., and Blackwell, B.: Interactions of monoamine oxidase inhibitors, amines and foodstuffs. *Adv Pharmacol Chemother* **8:** 185, 1970.
35. Marsden, C.D., Tarsy, D., and Baldessarni, R.J.: Spontaneous and drug induced movement disorders in psychotic patients. In *Psychiatric Complications of Neurological Diseases*, D.F. Benson and D. Blumer, Eds. Grune and Stratton, New York, 1975.
36. Martin, W.R., Sloan, J.W., Sapira, J.D., and Jasinski, D.R.: Physiologic, subjective and behavioral effects of amphetamine, methamphetamine, ephedrine, phenmetrazine and methylphenidat in man. *Clin Pharmacol Ther* **12:** 245, 1971.
37. Matter, B.J., Donat, P.E., Brill, M.L., and Ginn, H.F.: Tranylcypromine sulfate poisoning. *Arch Intern Med* **116:** 18, 1965.
38. Matthysse, S.: Antipsychotic drug actions: A clue to the neuropathology of schizophrenia. *Fed Proc* **32:** 200, 1975.
39. *Medical Letter* **18:** 74, 1970.
40. Millichap, J.G., and Fowler, G.W.: Treatment of "minimal brain dysfunction" syndromes. *Pediatr Clin North Am* **14:** 767, 1967.
41. Morselli, P.L., Principi, N., Tognoni, G., Reali, E., Belvedere, G., Standen, S.M., and Sereni, F.: Diazepam elimination in premature and full term infants and children. *J Perinat Med* **1:** 133, 1973.
42. Ney, P.G.: Psychosis in a child, associated with amphetamine administration. *Can Med Assoc J* **97:** 1026, 1967.
43. Poussaint, A.F., Ditman, K., and Greenfield, R.: Amitriptyline in childhood enuresis. *Clin Pharmacol Ther* **7:** 21, 1966.

44. Raskin, A.: Adverse reactions to phenelzine: Results of a nine-hospital depression study. *J Clin Pharmacol* **12:** 22, 1972.
45. Rivera-Calimlim, L., Castaneda, L., and Lasagna, L.: Effects of mode of management on plasma chlorpromazine in psychiatric patients. *Clin Pharmacol Ther* **14:** 978, 1973.
46. Safer, D., Allen, R., and Barr, E.: Depression of growth in hyperactive children on stimulant drugs. *N Engl J Med* **287:** 217, 1972.
47. Simeon, J., Saletu, B., Saletu, M., Itil, T.M., and Da Silva, J.: Thiothixene in childhood psychoses. Presented at the Third International Symposium on Phenothiazines, Rockville, Maryland, 1973.
48. Sjoqvist, F., Alexanderson, B., Asberg, M., Bertilsson, L., Borga, O., Hamberger, B., and Tuck, D.: Pharmacokinetics and biological effects of nortriptyline in man. *Acta Pharmacol Toxicol* **29** (Suppl. 3): 255, 1971.
49. Snyder, S.H.: How amphetamine acts in minimal brain dysfunction. *Ann NY Acad Sci* **205:** 310, 1973.
50. Thorstrand, C.: Cardiovascular effects of poisoning with tricyclic antidepressants. *Acta Med Scand* **195:** 205, 1974.
51. Winsberg, B.G., Perel, J., Hurivic, M., and Klutch, A.: Imipramine protein binding and pharmacokinetics in children. In *The Phenothiazines and Structurally Related Drugs*, I.S. Forrest, C.J. Carr and E. Usdin, Eds. New York, 1974.
52. Zingales, I.A.: A gas chromatographic method for the determination of haloperidol in human plasma. *J Chromatog* **54:** 15, 1971.

Appendix I

Guidelines for Psychostimulant Use

Until assay methods are developed for the psychostimulants generally used in MED, the following guidelines established by the American Academy of Pediatrics are recommended.[1]

1. Well-controlled studies employing a double-blind, crossover design and/or placebo drug are necessary. The absolute necessity of using a placebo is reinforced by study results, especially since the effects of one of the drugs under evaluation differed only slightly from the placebo.

2. The number of patients involved in a study should approximate 100. Too sparse a sampling impedes definite conclusions.

3. The psychological effect of being in a study (Hawthorne effect) must be considered. The stimulation produced by participation and the general effect of increased personal attention can result in an improvement unrelated to the effects of the drug.

4. Test situations which remove a patient from his general environment provide for a variable that often results in improvement.

5. Use of sensitive and precise diagnostic criteria would eliminate the possibility of undetected, underlying organic disease that might affect test results.

6. Discrimination between the organic and psychogenic effects produced by the drugs must be considered in establishing a study program.

7. Well-controlled investigations evaluating the influences of drugs on epileptic children, nonepileptic children, and children with normal and abnormal but not diagnostic EEG patterns need to be implemented.

8. There is need for focus on specific learning problems, with a corresponding identification of the influence of a drug on the specific symptom.

9. The potential adverse side effects of the drugs warrant more attention.

10. The variations in observational methods and lack of continuity in the observers result in incomparable data.

In summary, certain drugs have a promising effect on the treatment of children with learning impediments, but assessment of the true pharmacologic effect necessitates the accumulation of comparable, long-term, properly controlled studies and a careful evaluation of these data, compared alone and with adjunctive therapy.

Reference

1. Weiss, C.F., Yaffe, S.J., Cann, H.M., Gold, A.P., Kenny, F.M., Riley, H.D., Jr., Schafer, I., Stern, L., and Shirkey, H.C.: American Academy of Pediatrics Committee on Drugs, Guidelines on Psychostimulant Drugs. *Pediatrics* **46:** 142–144, 1970.

Appendix II

Some Drugs Used to Lessen Learning Impediments

Generic Name	*Trade Name*
Central Nervous System Stimulants	
Methylphenidate	Ritalin
Amphetamines	Dexedrine and Benzedrine
Deanol	Deaner
Pemoline	Cylert
Tranquilizing Agents	
Diazepam	Valium
Chlordiazepoxide	Librium
Chlorpromazine	Thorazine
Reserpine	Serpasil
Hydroxyzine	Atarax
Meprobamate	Miltown
Fluphenazine	Prolixin
Chlorprothixene	Taractan
Promazine	Sparine
Antihistaminics	
Phenothiazines	
Anticonvulsants	
Primidone	Mysoline
Diphenylhydantoin	Dilantin
Ethosuximide	Zarontin

3

Current Status of Medications for MBD

Lester F. Soyka

The purpose of this chapter is to develop a conceptual framework for evaluating the current status of drugs used for minimal brain dysfunction, based on a consideration of their possible mechanisms of action, from both a biochemical and a behavioral framework. It will cover the principal agents now in use: D-amphetamine (Dexedrine), methylphenidate (Ritalin), pemoline (Cylert), and the tricyclic antidepressants, of which imipramine (Tofranil) is the prototype.

To evaluate the current status of these drugs, we need to ask How do these drugs act? Where do they act? Are they all the same? If not, how can we choose the right drug for an individual patient? What directions might be taken for new drug development? Not all these questions can be answered definitely, but an attempt to do so can be made.

We will need to make certain assumptions. While any one of these can be criticized, we propose that they are reasonable assumptions and can form a basis from which to start. These assumptions are

Professor of Pharmacology and Pediatrics and Chairman, Department of Pharmacology, University of Vermont, Burlington, Vermont.

the following: (1) Currently employed agents *do* alter behavior in therapeutically useful ways; (2) patterns of behavior and particular behaviors arise from a complex interaction of neural and electrochemical events; (3) drug- and disease-induced alterations in biogenic amines of the brain cause alterations of behavior, levels of motor activity, hormonal homeostasis, mood states, etc.; and (4) analogies exist in the synthesis, transport, storage, release, etc., of biogenic amines in the peripheral adrenergic neuron and nerve terminals or synaptosomes of brain neurones.

I should begin by providing a overview of the commonly used drugs, reviewing each from the standpoint of its clinical pharmacology (Fig. 1).

Amphetamine is a phenylethylamine derivative, a structure common to most sympathomimetic drugs and many central nervous system stimulants. It will be discussed again in connection with the catecholamines. Amphetamine is the prototype central nervous system stimulant and the most widely investigated of this class of drugs. Chemically, it has an asymmetric alpha carbon so that it exists in a D and an L form, a point which has considerable importance (see below). The dextro form, or Dexedrine, is the most widely employed. Benzedrine is the racemic mixture of D and L. Though amphetamine has selective CNS stimulant properties, it does exhibit peripheral alpha and beta adrenergic actions, as is common with most other sympathomimetic drugs, especially in larger doses. The central nervous stimulant effects of amphetamine were used clinically as early as 1935 to treat narcolepsy.

Oral doses of amphetamine initially increase systolic blood pressure, and the heart rate is often reflexly slowed. Amphetamine affects all smooth muscles, with relaxation of the bronchial muscles and contraction of the urinary bladder sphincter.

CNS effects are on the cortex, spinal cord, reticular formation, and the respiratory center. In general, amphetamine accelerates and dsynchronizes the EEG.

Its acute toxic effects are clear extensions of its predictable pharmacologic effects. Addiction may occur and tolerance almost invariably develops, particularly with large doses, when the drug is used for mood improvement in psychiatric patients or when it is used as an appetite suppressant. Conversely in cases of narcolepsy and in MBD tolerance apparently does not develop.

Methamphetamine is closely related to amphetamine, differing only by the addition of a methyl group on the amine, and its pharmacologic actions are similar, but it has relatively more pronounced CNS effects, with little or no significant peripheral actions. To relate these

STRUCTURES OF CNS STIMULANTS

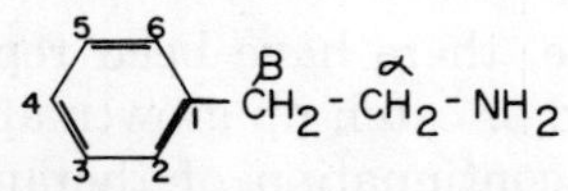

β-PHENYLETHYLAMINE

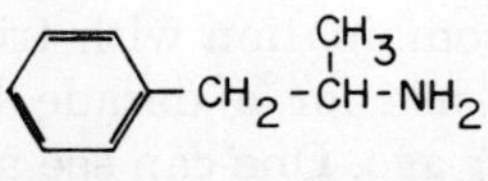

dl-AMPHETAMINE (BENZEDRINE)

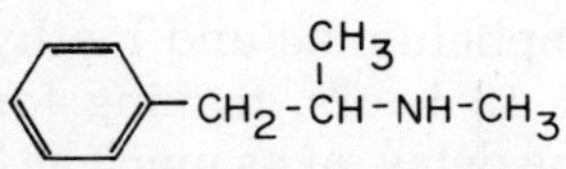

METHAMPHETAMINE (DESOXYN)

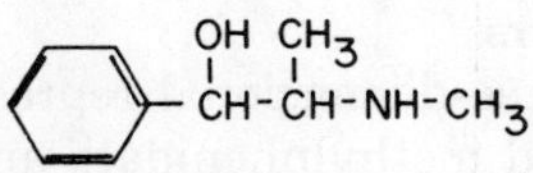

EPHEDRINE

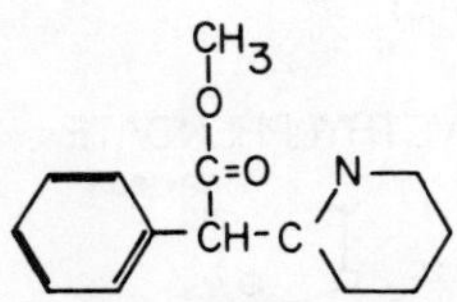

METHYLPHENIDATE (RITALIN)

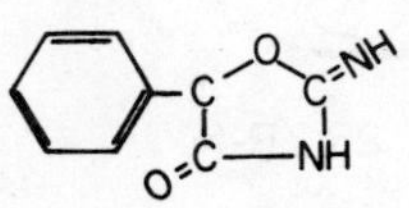

PEMOLINE (CYLERT)

Figure 1. Formulas of several CNS stimulants, illustrating their structural similarity and relationship to the fundamental phenylethylamine molecule.

structures, I have included ephedrine, which differs only in the presence of a hydroxyl group on the beta carbon (see above).

Methylphenidate is a piperidine derivative that is structurally related to amphetamine. With a little imagination one can see the basic phenylethylamine structure within. It is a mild CNS stimulant, with more prominent effects on mental than on motor activities, although large doses produce generalized CNS stimulation, which can lead to convulsions.

As with amphetamine, there have been reports of growth suppression, although rebound or catch-up growth appears to be the general pattern following discontinuation of therapy. High doses have also been reported to cause increases in heart rate. As is the case with amphetamine, methylphenidate is effective in the treatment of narcolepsy, either alone or in combination with tricyclic antirepressants.

Pemoline has been in use for a decade but was approved for marketing only about 1 year ago. One can see again the basic phenylethylamine structure and a certain resemblance to methylphenidate, so that it is not surprising that pemoline exhibits marked pharmacologic similarities to amphetamine and methylphenidate. Its serum half-life is longer, about 12 hours, making for some convenience of dosing. Unexplained is the delay, of as much as 3–4 weeks, in the onset of therapeutic effects, which is in sharp contrast to the nearly immediate onset with the other agents. Insomnia is the chief side-effect, though anorexia also occurs.

Figure 2 shows a three-dimensional representation of the structures of amphetamine and methylphenidate and illustrates the basic relationship of amphetamine and methylphenidate to beta-phenylethylamine and to one another. I shall describe below a membrane

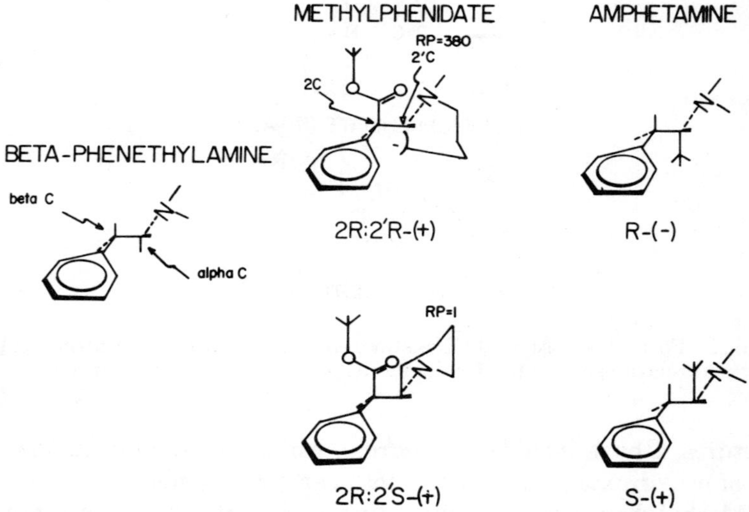

Figure 2. Three-dimensional representation of the methylphenidate and amphetamine molecules, illustrating their similarity to one another, and their close relationship to the structure of phenylethylamine. From Ferris, Tang and Maxwell.[2B]

"pump" which appears to recognize the phenylethylamine end of these molecules, leading to analogies in their actions.

Imipramine (Tofranil) is the prototype of the tricyclic antidepressants (Fig. 3). There are many examples in this class. Desimipramine is the principal and probably the active metabolite formed by *N*-demethylation of imipramine in the liver.

The structures of these compounds suggest important interrelationships of pharmacologic effects. For example, imipramine and promazine, a phenothiazine marketed as Sparine, are identical except for an ethylene bridge in the center ring in place of a sulfur atom. Desimipramine differs from imipramine by an *N*-demethylation, a reaction which is typical of hepatic drug metabolism. Amitriptyline (Elavil) has a carbon substituted for nitrogen in the central ring and the side chain is attached by a double bond. This is analogous to the conversion of a phenothiazine to a thioxanthene—drugs commonly used for major mental illnesses. Examples of such conversions would be chlorprothixene (Taractan) and thiothixene (Narvane). Thus one can see that close chemical relationships exist between the so-called major tranquilizers, the antipsychotic drugs, and the tricyclic antidepressants. Again, we find amitriptyline marketed as it's demethylated derivative nortriptyline (see also doxepin).

The tricyclics are frequently used in adults with a variety of behavioral manifestations as well as in depressed patients. In the doses found to be therapeutic in depressed patients these drugs are unique in their *lack* of apparent behavioral effects on animals or normal subjcts. In contrast to the usual *2–3-week delay* in the onset of action of imipramine when used to treat depression, some clinicians have observed that there is a *rapid* "on–off" effect of imipramine in

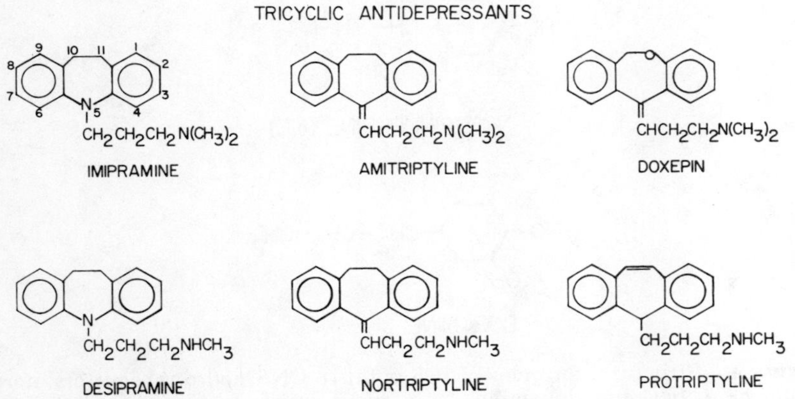

Figure 3. Structural formulas of commonly used tricyclic antidepressants.

patients with MBD. Curiously, this is also true of its use in enuresis. This is in contrast to the delayed onset of action of pemoline, as mentioned previously.

In order to understand the possible mechanisms of action of drugs commonly used to treat hyperkinesis, it is essential to be familiar with current concepts of the structure and function of the noradrenergic and dopaminergic neurons. Data have been obtained largely from studies of peripheral norepinephrine (NE) containing neurons (e.g., in the heart and blood vessels); however, essentially all data obtained from brain slices and synaptosome preparations are consistent with the major data from the peripheral nervous system.

Figure 4 again shows the basic phenylethylamine structure.

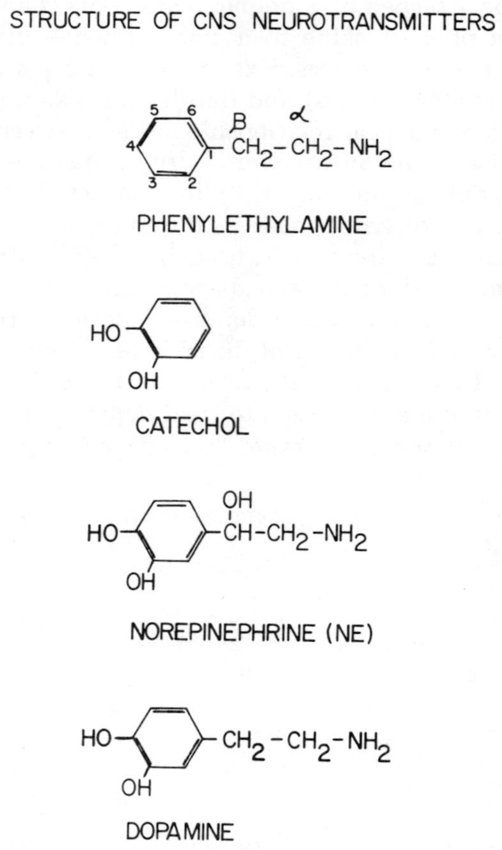

Figure 4. Structural formulas of two putative CNS neurotransmitters, norepinephrine (NE) and dopamine. Note the relation to the phenylethylamine nucleus and to the catechol structure.

When two hydroxyl groups are on the phenyl ring, in the 3 and 4 positions, the derivatives are termed *catechols*; thus norepinephrine and dopamine are termed *catecholamines*. There are other putative neurotransmitters, particularly serotonin (5-hydroxytryptamine) and gamma-aminobutyric acid (GABA), but relatively little is known of their relation to the drugs under discussion.

Synthesis of catecholamine neurotransmitters occurs *in situ* intraneuronally in the CNS (Fig. 5). The amino acid *tyrosine* is taken up from the blood stream and ring-hydroxylated to dopa in the cytoplasm of the neuron. The enzyme catalyzing this step is tyrosine hydroxylase. This hydroxylation is thought to be the rate-limiting step in the synthesis of the catecholamines, dopamine (DA), and norepinephrine (NE). Thus inhibition of tyrosine hydroxylase results in a decline of CNS NE and DA levels; this does not occur after partial inhibition of the other enzymes in the pathway. Dopa is then decarboxylated in the cytoplasm of the cell by dopa-decarboxylase, and DA is formed. DA is then transported into storage granules and hydroxylated in the beta position by the enzyme dopamine beta-hydroxylase, which is localized on the membrane of the storage granules.

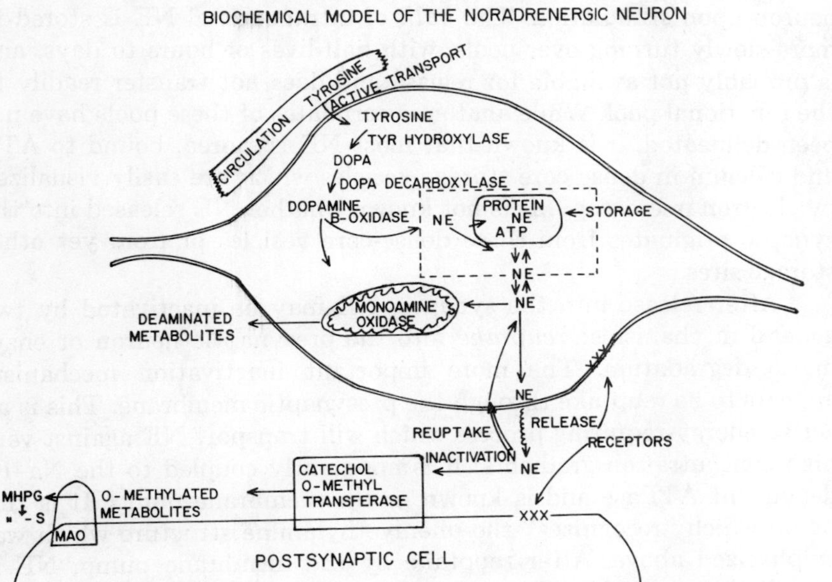

Figure 5. Schema of reactions occurring in the nerve terminals of noradrenergic neurones. MHPG = 3-methoxy-4-hydroxy phenylglycol. MHPG-S = 3-methoxy-4-hydroxy phenylglycol sulfate. From Cooper, Bloom, and Roth (1977).

The rate of synthesis of NE is variable and apparently controlled by a process known as feedback inhibition. The activity of the rate-limiting enzyme, tyrosine hydroxylase, is modulated by the intraneuronal NE concentration. High intraneuronal NE concentrations inhibit the activity of this enzyme, and thereby slow synthesis of NE; low intraneuronal NE concentrations, secondary to release of transmitter by physiologic stimuli or to drug action, increases the activity of tyrosine hydroxylase. To summarize, synthesis of transmitter occurs in nerve and is subject to regulation by the end products of the synthetic pathway. Thus, the rate of synthesis of NE is dependent on the rate of turnover of NE, where turnover is defined as the rate of utilization of the neurotransmitter. Another control mechanism recently described is exerted via presynaptic receptors.

The storage and release of CA transmitters is a complex phenomenon not completely understood. Brain NE is compartmentalized into a number of *functional* intraneuronal storage sites, each having a different half-life; three such storage pools have been described. NE turnover in the so-called functional pool is quite rapid, with a half-life of only 20 minutes. This relatively small, rapidly turning over pool, is very important to physiologic function, for it appears to represent *newly synthesized* NE, which is *preferentially* released from the neuron upon stimulation. The *bulk* of intraneuronal NE is stored in more slowly turning over pools, with half-lives of hours to days, and is probably not available for release and does not transfer readily to the functional pool. While anatomic correlates of these pools have not been delineated, it is known that most NE is stored, bound to ATP and calcium in dense-core storage vesicles which are easily visualized by electron microscopy. It is not known whether NE released into the synapse originates from these dense-core vesicles or from yet other storage sites.

After release into the synapse, NE may be inactivated by two general mechanisms: *reuptake* into the presynaptic neuron or enzymatic degradation. The more important inactivation mechanism appears to be reuptake through the presynaptic membrane. This is an active energy-requiring process which will transport NE against very high concentration gradients; it is apparently coupled to the Na–K-dependent ATPase and is known as the membrane pump. It is this pump which "recognizes" the phenlyethylamine structure which was emphasized above. After reuptake by the membrane pump, NE is rapidly deaminated by the enzyme *monoamine oxidase* (MAO), which is present in the mitochondria of the presynaptic neuron. Another enzyme, catechol-O-methyl transferase (COMT), is bound to the postsynaptic membrane, and may O-methylate and deactivate NE present in the synaptic cleft. It is thought that COMT does not play a major role in NE inactivation since inhibition of this enzyme does not significantly potentiate the effects of nerve stimulation.

With a schematic model of a central noradrenergic neuron, we can consider a number of drugs which interefere, or interact, with this system (Fig. 6). First there is alpha-methyltyrosine, which inhibits the hydroxylation of tyrosine by tyrosine hydroxylase. The uptake of tyrosine is relatively non-specific, and other amino acids will be taken into the neuron. Because of their usual low serum level they do not interefere with this process. One prominent exception is in *phenylketonuria,* in which the high levels of phenylalanine compete with tyrosine. This is believed by some to be related to the brain dysfunction in this disorder. The proposed role for nutrients in MBD has focused on the relatively non-specific nature of the amino acid uptake pump.

Reserpine interferes with the transport and storage mechanism of the granules. The depletion of norepinephrine produced by reserpine is long lasting, since the storage granules are irreversibly damaged.

Drugs which release norepinephrine are called indirect-acting agonists, of which amphetamine and ephedrine are examples. Am-

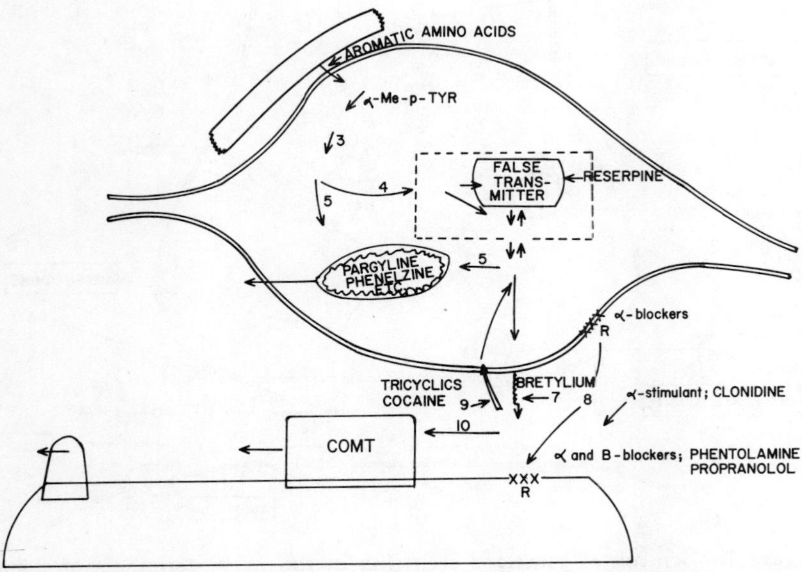

Figure 6. Site of action of drugs acting on noradrenergic transmission in the CNS. α-Me-p-TYR = alpha-methyl-p-tyrosine; R = receptor; COMT = catechol-O-methyltransferase. From Cooper, Bloom, and Roth.[1B]

phetamine, particularly the D-isomer, also acts directly to inhibit uptake, and therefore is called a mixed agonist. The pump mechanism for reuptake is also inhibited by the tricyclic antidepressants, of which desipramine is the model compound.

The MAO inhibitors act to prevent intraneuronal destruction of norepinephrine, as well as degradation of norepinephrine released into the synaptic cleft.

More selective CNS receptor–stimulating drugs are being developed. Currently the drug clonidine (Catapres) is an example of a central alpha adrenergic stimulant. It is proposed that, in certain areas of the brain, drug stimulation of receptors might have the same effect as release of norepinephrine or other neurotransmitters from the presynaptic terminal.

An analogous scheme is proposed for dopaminergic neurons in the central nervous system (Fig. 7). Tyrosine again is selectively taken up into the neuron and hydroxylated to dopa, which is converted to dopamine. This is taken up and stored in granules, analogous to the

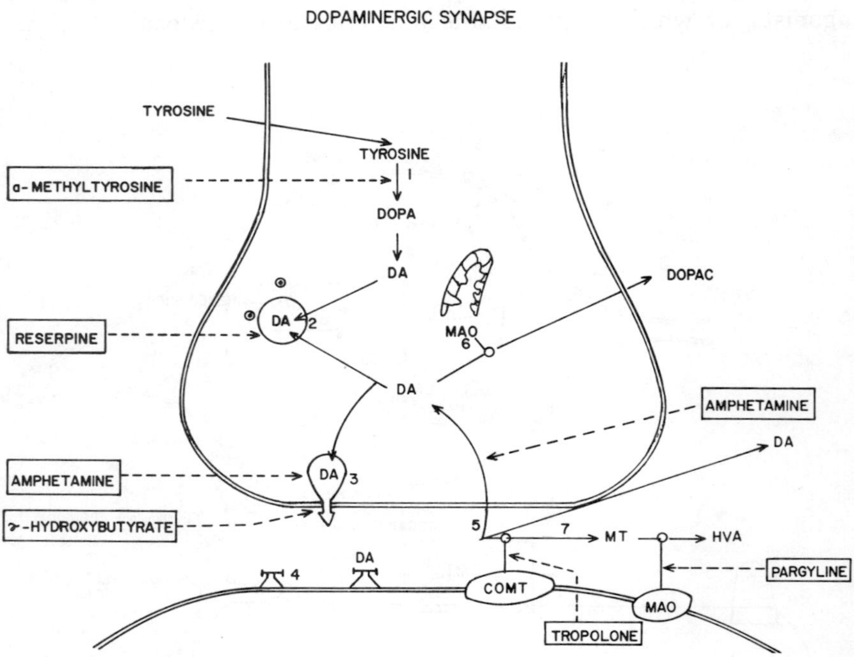

Figure 7. Schema of reactions occurring in the nerve terminals of dopaminergic neurones. DA = dopamine; DOPA = dihydroxyphenylalanine; MAO = monoamine oxidase; DOPAC = 3,4-dihydroxyphenyl acetic acid. MT = methyltyrosine; HVA = homovanillic acid. From Cooper, Bloom, and Roth.[1B]

storage granules for norepinephrine. Dopamine is then released, on nervous stimulation, into the synaptic cleft. Its actions are terminated by reuptake into the neuron, or by degradation by catechol-O-methyltransferase (COMT) localized outside the presynaptic neuron.

Drugs affecting the dopaminergic system are analogous to those affecting the noradrenergic system. Alpha-methyl-*p*-tyrosine is a potent inhibitor of tyrosine hydroxylase and decreases the amount of dopamine formed. Again, reserpine interferes with the uptake-storage mechanism of the granules. Amphetamine releases dopamine, analogous to the release of norepinephrine, and also inhibits its uptake. In contrast to the noradrenergic neuron, the reuptake of dopamine is *not* inhibited to a significant extent by the tricyclics.

Several direct-acting stimulants are known. The most obvious is levodopa, which is converted in the brain to dopamine. Apomorphine, an analogue of morphine, is an effective dopamine receptor–stimulating drug, and has been used to treat Parkinson's disease. Blockers of the dopamine receptor are also known; for example, perphenazine (Trilafon) is a piperazinyl phenothiazine used for psychoses and for control of severe nausea and vomiting. Haloperidol (Haldol) is a butyrophenone used in the management of psychotic disorders and for the control of tics and vocal utterances seen in the Gilles de la Tourette syndrome.

One of the most interesting papers in the field is that of Snyder and Meyerhoff, presented at a meeting of the New York Academy of Science on MBD in 1972 and titled "How amphetamine works in MBD." The paper was based on studies comparing the release of norepinephrine and of dopamine and the inhibition of their uptake by the two stereoisomers of amphetamine. As noted previously, amphetamine is a racemic mixture when sold as Benezedrine. The D isomer, the more potent CNS stimulant and also the most widely used, is sold as Dexedrine.

Studies in Synder's laboratory indicated that the D isomer was more potent than the L isomer in inhibiting norepinephrine uptake, but that they were equally potent in inhibiting the uptake of dopamine. Similarly, D-amphetamine was a more potent releaser of norepinephrine, whereas the two isomers were equally potent in causing release of dopamine. Based on these observations, one would propose that if D-amphetamine is more potent than the L form in eliciting a particular effect, norepinephrine may be responsible. Whereas if D and L isomers are equipotent, dopamine may be implicated (Table 1). In animals, amphetamine causes two characteristic effects: (1) an increase in motor activity, or hyperactivity; and (2) *stereotypy*, in which the animals perform repeated purposeless movements such as

TABLE 1
Differential Actions of Amphetamine Isomers

Neurochemical Effect	*Isomer Activity*
Inhibition of norepinephrine (NE) reuptake	D > L
Inhibition of dopamine reuptake	D ~ L
Release of NE	D >> L
Release of dopamine	D ~ L

Therefore, if D-amphetamine more potent than L- in eliciting an effect, NE involved; if D~L, then dopamine implicated.

Based on this hypothesis:

Species	*Behavior*	*Neurotransmitter Responsible*
Rat	Motor hyperactivity	NE
	Stereotypy	Dopamine
Man	Hyperactivity	Dopamine
	Amphetamine psychosis	Dopamine

The top portion indicates the relative activity determined from *in vitro* studies, chiefly of rat brain. The lower portion relates these actions to behavioral observations in rat and man. Adapted from Snyder and Meyerhoff.[5B]

gnawing, grooming, and chewing. Snyder and co-workers found that D-amphetamine was 10 times more potent than the L isomer in increasing motor activity, and concluded therefore that norepinephrine was involved in this action. Whereas for stereotypy, the D form was only twice as potent as the L form, suggesting that dopamine was playing a major role.

In humans, amphetamine is known to produce acute psychosis, and in this effect the D and L isomers are equally active; by analogy, then, it was proposed that dopamine was involved in this effect.

Synder and Meyerhoff presented data from studies of an 8-year-old girl with Gilles de la Tourette's disease accompanied by classic MBD. This is an unusual syndrome of body tics and barking noises, which develop into coprolalia, usaully beginning in childhood. During several months in a clinical research center, the patient was administered either D- or L-amphetamine. D-amphetamine produced marked exacerbation of the tic, whereas L-amphetamine had little effect. Snyder and Meyerhoff therefore postulated that norepinephrine was responsible for the tics. The patients hyperactivity responded equally well to both isomers, suggesting that dopamine was involved. There is some anatomic support for this proposal, in that the septal areas of the brain are believed to be involved in emotionality and are rich in norepinephrine, whereas the corpus striatum is rich in dopamine and is involved in motor activity. These provocative observations need be tempered, since the drugs may act in several areas of the brain and the drug response may not necessarily be related to the underlying cause. This obviously is a particular problem with MBD, the pathophysiology of which is insufficiently known.

Janowsky and Davis examined drug affects in schizophrenic patients and found that L-dopa aggravated schizophrenia, D-Amphetamine worsened psychotic symptoms, but was less potent than methylphenidate. L-Amphetamine was the least potent of the three. Angrist and co-workers administered amphetamine to former amphetamine addicts and found that D-amphetamine was twice as potent as the L isomer in causing psychosis. These studies are more or less in keeping with the results of Snyder's findings with stereotypy in animals.

Ferris, Tang, and Maxwell studied methylphenidate in comparison with the isomers of amphetamine and concluded that methylphenidate is a selective, central dopamine releaser. Thus several lines of investigation suggest that *dopaminergic* neurons are involved in hyperkinesis.

Our primitive state of knowledge in this area may be analogous to the biogenic amine theory of depression. Here a simple hypothesis, consistent with a variety of drug responses has been proposed, yet the vast amount of conflicting data, and the complex nature of the problem itself, makes one hesitant about accepting such simplistic theories. Nonetheless, it is clear that such proposals are a great stimulant to further investigation.

Another class of drugs that deserves brief mention are the monoamine oxidase inhibitors. We have seen that monoamine oxidase is an important enzyme for the degradation of both norepinephrine and dopamine. Huessy and others have reported that inhibitors of monoamine oxidase may be useful in the treatment of children with MBD. One of the monoamine oxidase inhibitors that we have found to be particularly interesting is tranylcypromine (Parnate) (Fig. 8).

This is a non-hydrazine MAO inhibitor with a rapid onset of activity. Its structure is strikingly similar to that of ampetamine, with the side chain in a ring. This compound increases the concentration of epinephrine, norepinephrine, and serotonin in storage sites throughout the nervous system, and it is proposed that this increased concentration in the brain stem is the basis for its antidepressant activity. The structural similarity of many of the compounds used for treating psychiatric illnesses, depression, schizophrenia, and MBD is striking.

Table 2 summarizes the current theoretical conceptual relationship between the more commonly used drugs in hyperkinesis and MBD, and their effects on the dopamine-norepinephrine system.

Let us now turn to consideration of drug action from the behavioral point of view. I am indebted to my colleague, A. Bruce Campbell,

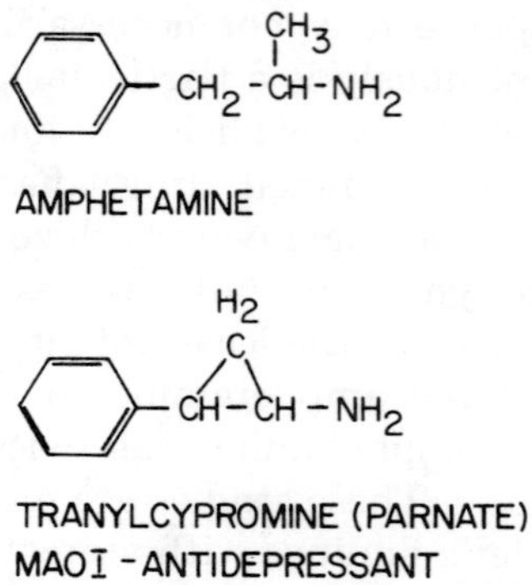

Figure 8. Formula of tranylcypromine. Note its close structural resemblance to amphetamine.

Ph.D., M.D., for his assistance in the preparation of this section, and it is largely his work that is presented here.

Much current research in psychopharmacology is based on observations of drug effects in a specific behavioral paradigm originated by B. F. Skinner, which is known as operant, or instrumental, conditioning. Skinner's original contention was that the mammalian central nervous system, especially as regards behavior, was too complex to allow "reductionist" investigation (i.e., lesion making, stimulation, and other surgical/chemical procedures) into the neural substrates of behavior. Alternatively, he proposed that the organism be considered a "black box," and that behavior is definable and predictable solely in terms of the effect of a precise environmental manipulation on behavior. That is, Skinner strove to develop an *operational* definition of the relationship between the environment and behavior, and not a theoretical explanation of how neural systems resulted in behavior. Since Skinner's pioneering work, technology has been developed which has permitted investigation of the neural mechanisms mediating behav-

TABLE 2
Summary of Principal Neurochemical Actions of Drugs Used to Treat MBD

D,L-amphetamine	Inhibits reuptake of dopamine Releases dopamine
D-amphetamine	Inhibits reuptake of NE Releases NE
Pemoline	Increases rate of synthesis of dopamine
Tricyclic antidepressants	Inhibit uptake of NE
Methylphenidate	Inhibits uptake of NE

ioral responses to environmental changes, including drug administration. Such work is now the frontier of neuropsychopharmacology, and some data from this field offer interesting insights into what has been called the *paradoxical* action of stimulant drugs in hyperkinesis.

The operant paradigm is simple; it involves the presentation or removal of a rewarding or punishing stimulus, contingent on the performance of a specific response by the organism. The classic example is a pigeon pecking a key to obtain food. This paradigm is termed *positive reinforcement* and may be written in shorthand as $R \rightarrow S^{R+}$ where *R* represents the response, and S^{R+} represents a rewarding, or positively reinforcing, stimulus. A positively reinforcing stimulus is operationally defined as any stimulus that, when elicited by a response, results in an increased probability, or rate of occurrence, of that response.

There are four operant paradigms (Table 3).

1. Positive reinforcement, as described above.
2. Negative reinforcement, in which performance of a response results in removal of an aversive stimulus (i.e., bar pressing to turn off an electric shock).
3. Punishment, in which performance of a response elicits an aversive stimulus, and the response rate therefore declines.
4. Extinction, in which performance of a response that was previously reinforced no longer elicits that stimulus.

It should be noted that both positive *and* negative reinforcement result in an increased response rate, and that *negative reinforcement* and *punishment* are *not* interchangable terms. Most of the experiments to be described utilize either positive or negative reinforcement.

One characteristic of operant behavior is that it can be differentiated in form and temporal patterning by contingent events or reinforcers. Since the act of reinforcement is the presentation of a reinforcer in a specified temporal relationship to a response (operant), this temporal relationship has been shown to dictate the pattern and

TABLE 3
Summary of Four Possible Operant Paradigms

	Types of Conditioning	
Rate	*Contingency: Stimulus Presented*	*Contingency: Stimulus Removed, Absent, or Avoided*
Increased	1. "Positive Reinforcement"	2. "Negative Reinforcement"
Decreased	3. "Punishment"	4. "Extinction"

rate of responding reliably and reproducibly. The exact temporal relationship between the response and the reinforcer is termed the *schedule of reinforcement.* The simplest schedule is continuous reinforcement (CRF), in which each response is followed by reinforcement. Simple, or first order, schedules may be divided into ratio and interval types. Each subtype may be divided into *fixed* or *variable* classifications. In a ratio schedule, a response is reinforced after the performance of a designated number of responses; the number required may be fixed or variable. For instance, if every tenth response is reinforced, the schedule is FR 10; if the number of responses required ranges between 5 and 15, but averages 10, the schedule is VR 10. In interval schedules, reinforcement is available after some designated period has passed since the previous reinforcement, irrespective of the number of responses that have occurred; the time interval may be either fixed or variable. For example, in an FI 30 second (FI 30″) schedule, the next response occurring 30 seconds after the previous reinforcement has passed will be reinforced. A VI 30″ schedule is one in which the interreinforcement interval varies, but averages 30 seconds (Table 4).

Each type of schedule generates a characteristic pattern of response that is the same regardless of the species of animal used. FR schedules usually generate continuous high rates of responding, with the response rate directly proportional to the ratio; however, the ratio can be increased to the point where very low response rates occur. VR and VI schedules elicit a continuous intermediate response immediately after reinforcement, which increases exponentially as the interval progresses, with very high response rates at the end of the interval, just prior to reinforcement.

The operant paradigm offers a number of advantages for the analysis of the behavioral effects of drugs. First, because the subject is in a closed environment, one can control nearly all aspects of the surroundings and minimize the effect of extraneous variables. Second,

TABLE 4
Typical Schedules Used for Reinforcement in Conditioning Experiments

Schedules of Reinforcement

1. Continuous Reinforcement (CRF)
2. Ratio Schedules
   - A. Fixed ratio (FR) (example, FR 10)
   - B. Variable ratio (VR) (example, VR 10)
3. Interval Schedules
   - A. Fixed interval (FI) (example, F 30″)
   - B. Variable interval (VI) (example, VI 30″)

one can control the rate and pattern of behavior through manipulation of schedule contingencies. Third, the behavior is easily measured and quantified, and does not require subjective interpretation.

In behavioral terms, any drug which increases the rate of occurrence of a behavior is termed a psychomotor stimulant. Nevertheless, psychomotor stimulants are probably the most frequently used class of drugs in the treatment of hyperkinesis, thus leading to labeling the effect of psychomotor stimulants in hyperkinetic children as paradoxical. The effect of these agents may be explicable on the basis of a phenomenon termed *drug-behavior interaction* by Seiden and Campbell (1974). They suggested that the effect of a drug on behavior is not simply dependent on the class of drug administered, but rather on a complex interaction of environmental contingencies, ongoing behavior, and the neurochemical state of the organism (Fig. 9).

The concept that the effect of a class of drugs might be at least partially dependent on the baseline rate of behavior was first proposed in 1955. Dews trained pigeons to peck for food on two different schedules of reinforcement: An FI 15′ schedule, which resulted in low response rates, and and FR 50, which resulted in high response rates. Both experimental groups were then given equivalent doses of pentobarbital, a barbiturate sedative. The drug caused a *decrease* in response rate on the FI 15′ schedule, but an *increase* in response rate on the FR 50 schedule. That is, a drug traditionally considered to be a depressant resulted in a decrease in rate of a "slow" behavior, and an increase in rate of a "fast" behavior! This observation led to the concept of *rate-dependent drug effect*. That is, the effect of a drug on a behavior may depend on the ongoing rate of that behavior at the time of drug administration.

Dews[4C] extended these observations to psychomotor stimulants. He studied the effects of methamphetamine on behavior maintained

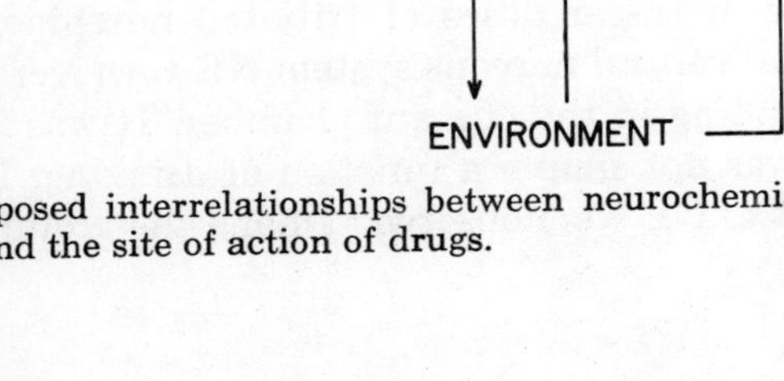

Figure 9. Proposed interrelationships between neurochemistry, behavior, and environment, and the site of action of drugs.

by four different schedules of food reinforcement. Two schedules elicited relatively high rates of responding (VI 1′ and FR 50); increasing doses of methamphetamine resulted in a progressive *decrease* in response rate on these schedules. The other two schedules (FI 15′ and FR 900) resulted in low response rates in the non-drug condition; when methamphetamine was administered to these animals, marked *increases* in rate of responding was observed. Dews's findings have been confirmed by several investigators using rats and primates. For instance, Kelleher and Morse (1964), using squirrel monkeys in a negative reinforcement paradigm, demonstrated that D-amphetamine increased low rates of responding on FI schedules, but *decreased* high rates of responding on FR schedules. The analogy to hyperkinetic children having high baseline rates of behavior to this rate-dependent drug effect is obvious.

Factors other than ongoing rate of behavior may determine the effect of psychomotor stimulants on response rate. Campbell and Seiden [3C] trained three groups of rats to press a bar for water on a VI 20″ schedule of reinforcement; this schedule engendered a relatively high response rate. Each group of animals received a different magnitude of reinforcement: 0.01 ml, 0.04 ml, or 0.10 ml. The control response rate of all three groups of animals was identical. However, D-amphetamine had little effect on the response rate of those animals responding for the largest amount of water. Amphetamine exerted a potent *rate-depressant effect* on those animals responding for small amounts of water. Thus, even when baseline response rates are similar, amphetamine may exert *differential* effects on behavior, apparently dependent on the *strength of reinforcement*. One can only speculate on the strength of reinforcement of various parental, school, and other influences acting as reinforcers. The magnitude of reinforcement maintaining hyperkinetic behavior is unknown. It is conceivable that reinforcement maintaining hyperkinetic behavior differs from that maintaining "normal" behavior, this being another determinant of amphetamine's effect in children. At any rate, the effect of psychomotor stimulants in hyperkinesis is entirely consistent with the observed action of amphetamine in several species of animals.

The neuropharmacologic basis of drug-behavior interactions observed with psychomotor stimulants is less clear. Lewy and Seiden (1972) trained rats to press a bar for water on a VI 30″ schedule. Through the use of tracer doses of tritiated norepinephrine it was demonstrated that central nervous system NE turnover was increased in animals responding in the operant chamber. It was further shown that this effect was not simply a function of drinking. No differences in absolute levels of NE were observed among the groups.

Schoenfeld and Seiden[9C] trained rats to press a level on an FR 10 schedule, and administered α-methyl-p-tyrosine, which is an inhibitor of tyrosine hydroxylase (see above). It was found that α-MT produced a large *decrease* in response rate on this schedule. Animals were then given L-dopa in varying doses, to enable *de novo* synthesis of transmitter after pretreatment with a-MT. It was found that the rate of response on the FR 10 schedule was directly proportional to the dose of L-dopa given. One can conclude from these data that the rate of response is directly proportional to the amount of transmitter, NE or DA, available for release. Thus, animals responding at different rates probably have different rates of catecholamine turnover. Campbell and Seiden[3C] demonstrated that even when response rates are equivalent, reinforcement *magnitude* may affect catecholamine turnover in the pons-medulla and thalamus than do animals responding for small amounts of water. Thus, behavioral states of environmental contingencies which result in rate-depressant amphetamine effects are associated with high rates of endogenous catecholamine turnover.

The relevance of this observation to the mechanism of amphetamine's rate-depressant effect is not entirely clear. However, amphetamine both increases release of catecholamines and prevents transmitter inactivation by blocking reuptake at the presynaptic membrane. Campbell and Seiden[3C] have postulated that the combined effect of very high rates of transmitter release, due to amphetamine and schedule or rate effect, and prevention of inactivation of transmitter by blockade of reuptake may result in a deplolarization block at key synaptic sites in the CNS and produce a net *depressant* effect on behavior. It is interesting that tricyclic antidepressants, which block transmitter reuptake, also have been observed to have rate-depressant effects in some behavioral experiments. Extrapolation of the above hypothesis to the hyperkinetic state in humans is obviously premature. Thus, the behavioral approach has given us two interesting and probably relevant notions about the action of drugs in MBD: (1) that the drug effect may be dependent on the rate of a particular behavior occurring at the time of drug administration, and (2) that the strength or magnitude of reinforcement can determine whether a psychomotor stimulant will cause an increase or a decrease in a particular behavior.

References

A. Drug Therapy of MBD

1. Baldessarini, R.J.: Pharmacology of amphetamines. *Pediatrics* **49**: 694–701, 1972.

2. Commentary, Committee on Drugs, American Academy of Pediatrics: Use of D-amphetamine and related central nervous system stimulants in children. *Pediatrics* **51:** 302–305, 1973.
3. Conners, C.K.: Psychological effects of stimulant drugs on children with minimal brain dysfunction. *Pediatrics* **49:** 702–704, 1972.
4. Eisenberg, L.: Clinical use of stimulant drugs in children. *Pediatrics* **49:** 709–715, 1972.
5. Gross, M.D.: Growth of hyperkinetic children taking methylphenidate, dextroamphetamine, or imipramine/desipramine. *Pediatrics* **58:** 423–431, 1976.
6. Huessy, H.R.: Minimal brain dysfunction in children: Recognition and treatment. *Drug Ther* **3:** 52–63, 1973.
7. Huessy, H.R.: Study of the prevalence and therapy of choreatiform syndrome or hyperkinesis in rural Vermont. *Acta Paedopsychiat* **34:** 130–135, 1967.
8. Medical Letter. Methylphenidate (Ritalin) and other drugs for treatment of hyperactive children. **19:** No. 13, 1977.
9. Oettinger, L.: Learning disorders, hyperkinesis and the use of drugs in children. *Rehabil Lit* **32:** 162–170, 1971.
10. Safer, D., Allen, R., and Barr, E.: Depression of growth in hyperactive children on stimulant drugs. *New Engl J Med* **287:** 217–220, 1972.
11. Sroufe, L.A., and Stewart, M.A.: Treating problem children with stimulant drugs. *New Engl J Med* **289:** 407–412, 1973.
12. Sulzbacher, S.I.: Psychotropic medication with children: An evaluation of procedural biases in results of reported studies. *Pediatrics* **51:** 513–517, 1973.

B. Neuropharmacology

1. Cooper, J.R., Bloom, F.E., and Roth, R.H. (Eds.): *The Biochemical Basis of Neuropharmacology* (3rd ed.), Oxford University Press, New York, 1977.
2. Ferris, R.M., Tang, F.L.M., and Maxwell, R.A.: A comparison of the capacities of isomers of amphetamine, deoxypipradrol and methylphenidate to inhibit the uptake of tritiated catecholamines in rat cerebral cortex slices, synaptosomal preparations of rat cerebral cortex, hypothalamus and striatum and into adrenergic nerves of rabbit aorta. *J Pharmacol Exp Ther* **181:** 407–416, 1972.
3. Iverson, L.L.: *The Uptake and Storage of Noradrenaline in Sympathetic Nerves.* Cambridge University Press, 1967.
4. Iverson, L.L.: Uptake mechanisms for neurotransmitter amines. *Biochem Pharmacol* **23:** 1927–1935, 1974.
5. Snyder, S.H., and Meyerhoff, J.L.: How amphetamine acts in minimal brain dysfunction. *Ann NY Acad Sci* **205:** 310–320, 1973.

C. Behavioral Pharmacology

1. Barchas, J.D., Akil, H., Elliott, G.R., Holman, R.B., and Watson, S.J.: Behavioral neurochemistry: Neuroregulators and behavioral states. *Science* **200:** 964–973, 1978.
2. Campbell, A.B., Brown, R.M., and Seiden, L.S.: A selective effect of p-chlorophenylalanine on fixed-ratio responding. *Physiol Behav* **7:** 853–857, 1971.
3. Campbell, A.B., and Seiden, L.S.: The effect of relative and absolute reinforcement magnitude on operant responding. *Physiol Behav* **12:** 843–849, 1974.

4. Dews, P.B.: Studies on behavior. IV. Stimulant actions of methamphetamine. *J Pharmacol Exp Ther* **122:** 137-147, 1958.
5. Kosman, M.E., and Unna, K.R.: Effects of chronic administration of the amphetamines and other stimulants on behavior. *Clin Pharmacol Ther* **9:** 240–254, 1968.
6. Lewy, A.J., and Seiden, L.S.: Operant behavior changes norepinephrine metabolism in rat brain. *Science* **175:** 454–456, 1971.
7. Lipton, M.A., DiMascio, A., and Killam, K.F. (Eds.): *Psychopharmacology: A Generation of Progress.* Raven Press, New York, 1978.
8. Martin, W.R., Sloan, J.W., Sapira, J.D., and Jasinski, D.R.: Physiologic, subjective and behavioral effects of amphetamine, methamphetamine, ephedrine, phenmetrazine and methylphenidate in man. *Clin Pharmacol Ther* **12:** 245–258, 1971.
9. Schoenfeld, R.I., and Seiden, L.S.: Effect of alpha-methyltyrosine on operant behavior and brain catecholamine levels. *J Pharmacol Exp Ther* **167:** 319–327, 1969.

4

Clinical Aspects of Minimal Brain Dysfunction: Diagnosis and Management

Eric Denhoff, M.D.

The criteria which identify children with minimal brain dysfunction (MBD) will be found in the history and the neurologic examination. Children with MBD have a history of adverse perinatal events. In one retrospective study the incidence was 32%.[1] Mothers of children with MBD have a similar background and obstetric history as mothers who later had neurologically impaired infants.[2] The profile of such mothers is outlined in Table 1.

In the histories of patients with MBD there is a high rate of family breakdown. Familial or genetic predisposition is found in 20–35% of cases. Mixed causes are the rule rather than the exception. In about 30% of cases no clear reasons will be found.[3]

In a controlled anterospective study a significant correlation was found between hyperreactive or hyporeactive behavior persisting to 1 year of age and failure in school at 7 years of age. The children who failed could be classified as having MBD. At birth some were premature or had hyperbilirubinemia or hemolytic disease. Others had respiratory distress syndrome. Seven years later these same children

---

Clinical Professor of Pediatrics, Brown University Program in Medicine, Providence, Rhode Island.

TABLE 1
Profile of a Mother Whose Baby Is at Risk for Later Neurologic Impairment

Sociological:	Divorced or separated, unmarried (age over 35 or under 16 years), less than high school education, excess smoking (three packs or more daily)
Illness:	Mental retardation, epilepsy, alcoholism and drugs, progressive neurologic disease, renal disease, rheumatic fever, asthma, thyroid disease
Pregnancy:	Placental disorders, hyperemesis gravida, hydramnios, cord prolapse, previous premature infants, reproductive difficulty, premature membrane rupture existing 12 hours or more
Delivery:	Breech and cesarean section, esepcially in a premature infant; high/mid forceps delivery

Mothers whose babies will have problems will have an abnormal incidence rate of two neurologically impaired babies per 1000 births (2%) or more, while mothers with normal babies will have a rate of less than one neurologically abnormal infant per 1000 births.
Data abstracted from Niswander and Gordon.[2]

failed screening tests which measured gross and fine motor skills, perceptual motor functioning, speech and language abilities, and school achievement.[4] This information is summarized in Table 2 and suggests that MBD children can be identified at as early as 1 year of age.

Neurologic Evaluation

A neurologic evaluation which is designed to detect involuntary movements and poor coordination is necessary for the diagnosis.[5] In a study of 48 children with MBD a high incidence of congenital stigmata was found as well as evidence of imbalance and adiadochokinesis as measured by bilateral finger skills and hand rotation patterns. Poor visual following of a moving target at 16 inches and difficulty in tongue placement were noted. A substantial number of these children were found to have deviations of the uvula (not as a result of tonsillectomy). Reflexes were frequently asymmetric, and extensor plantar reflexes were common. A few children had difficulty in pointing out objects or letters with the right hand when they identified the objects with the left (cross callosum dysfunction). Mixed dominance and laterality, and difficulty in distinguishing right from left, were common findings.[1] Table 3 provides guidelines for performing a neurologic evaluation which is useful in diagnosing MBD.

The average age of these children at examination was 9.6 years. At this age, normal neurologic capability is expected. Table 4 sum-

TABLE 2
Identification of MBD Children at 1 Year (N = 380)

First Year Outcome	*Causes in History*		*7-Year Status*	
Hyperreactivity	Respiratory distress syndrome	19%	WISC IQ	0.28[a]
Abnormal Moro reflex				
Excessive and persistent crying	Dysmaturity	6%	Wide Range Achievement	
Poor sucking and swallowing	Low birth weight	5%	Scores	0.20[b]
Hypertonia			Meeting Street School	
Abnormal jitteriness and tremulousness	Bilirubin level over 15 mg%	21%	Screening Test	0.38[b]
Asymmetric reflexes	Apgar at 5 minutes (6 or less)	22%		
Hyporreactivity				
Listless				
Lethargic				
Hypotonic-floppy				
Development				
Normal motor				
Delayed speech and language				

[a] $p = 0.05$ (one-tailed test).
[b] $p = 0.01$ (one-tailed test).

TABLE 3
Guidelines for Neurologic Evaluation[a]

TASK	TIME/sec	AGE/years	ANATOMIC CORRELATES AREA
I BALANCE-CO-ORDINATION			
ROMBERG	15		FRONTAL-CEREBELLAR-HYPOTHALAMIC
BALANCE, ONE FOOT	15	6-7½	
FINGER-NOSE	3 TIMES		
II CHOREIFORM MOVEMENTS			
FINGERS OUTSTRETCHED	5	5	DIENCEPHALIC-LIMBIC
	10	6-7	
	15	7-8	
	30	8+	
III DIADOCHOKINESIS	20 MVTS/10 sec	6-7½	FRONTAL-PRE-CENTRAL (MOTOR)
IV ORGANIZED MOVEMENTS			
WALK BACKWARDS	2 STEPS	3	
HEEL-TOE	6 feet	3½-5½	SAME
HOP; SKIP	6 feet	5-6	
V DIRECTIONALITY			FRONTAL-PRECENTRAL
RIGHT-LEFT	2	5-7½	
VI PATTERNED MOVEMENTS			
FINGER-THUMB, BILAT.	3	5	
FINGERS-THUMB, BILAT.	2	6-7½	SAME
OPEN-CLOSE MOUTH	5	6-7½	
VII ARTICULATION			FRONTAL-CEREBELLAR-TEMPORAL
Puh-Puh-Puh	2	5	
Puh-Kuh-Tuh	2	6-7½	
Tuh-Puh-Kuh	2	8	
VIII SENSORY INTEGRATION			
GRAPHESTHESIA	○, ×, □	5	POST-CENTRAL (SENSORY INTAKE)
	△ ◇	6-7½	
	1, 3, 6, 9		
STEREOGNOSIS	KEY		
	COINS	6-7½	
	BUTTONS		
	HUOVY	8+	
IX COMPLEX INTEGRATION			
FINGER COUNTING	2	6-7½	FRONTAL-CEREBELLAR
GNOSIA	2	6-7½	
X INTERSENSORY PROCESSING			
AUDITORY-MOTOR	2	6-7½	TEMPORAL-OCCIPITAL
VISUAL-MOTOR	2		

[a] Developed from Denhoff, E., et al.: Items from the meeting "Street School Screening Tests.": *Dev Med* **10:** 220, 1968.

TABLE 4
Key Findings on the Neurological Examination in MBD

Findings	*Per Cent*
Stigmata	
Hypertelorism; lowset ears	25
Widened gap between toes	
Gross and Fine Motor Skills	
Inability to balance 5 sec. or more on one foot	54
Poor finger-nose skills	18
Poor diadokinetic skills (finger, hand)	13
Cranial Nerves	
Inefficient visual following	41
Inefficient tongue movements	29
Deviated uvula	25
Deep Reflexes	
Asymmetric and increased	25
Plantars, extensor	18
Higher Cortical Processing	
Abnormal cross-callosum ability by stereognosis or graphesthesia	10
Body Organization Skills	
Poor differentiation of right and left	33
Mixed dominance and laterality	42
Poor position sense, fingers	18

marizes the key findings in 48 children with MBD.

Psychological and educational tests and the electroencephalogram are also used in diagnosis but they will not be discussed here.

Management

Management must be comprehensive and not limited solely to the use of psychostimulant medication. In each case a custom-designed educational program is necessary, as well as a behavior modification program. Child and family support services are also imperative in hard-core cases if a successful outcome is desired.

Psychostimulant Medication

Medication appears to benefit best the MBD child with a high risk perinatal–infancy profile, a cluster of atypical neurologic and/or psychological test findings, and an abnormal electroencephalogram, especially if there is poorly sustained alpha rhythm or interhemispheric asymmetry. Generally these findings occur in clusters rather than in isolation.

There are other types of MBD, such as those arising from acute head trauma or meningoencephalitis. These types respond less well to medication. Genetic types with few neurologic findings do not respond as well to medication.

There are some overactive children without MBD who respond well to psychostimulant medication for a short period. These are generally bright, highly verbal children who are undergoing great emotional stress due to family breakdown or school or peer group pressure.

Medication can be used to determine if a child will respond beneficially to a psychostimulant drug.[6]

A single 5-mg tablet of amphetamine sulfate or 10-mg methylphenidate will demonstrate action within a half hour after oral ingestion. It will reach a peak within 3–3½ hours, and be manifested as a measurably improved attention span. The effect will no longer be apparent at the end of 4–5 hours.

The effect of a single 5-mg tablet of dextroamphetamine sulfate on attention span can be measured by analyzing pre-drug and on-drug "on-task" behavior. The physician tests the child on a battery of standardized academic tasks, such as reading a paragraph or spelling grade-appropriate words. Measurably improved on-task performance within the hour suggests a beneficial medication effect. Table 5 is an example of an attention span rating form that is useful in clinical practice.

If on-task behavior shows no change on dextroamphetamine, then a single 10-mg tablet of levo-amphetamine (Benzedrine) sulfate on another day is substituted, and the test procedures are repeated. Improvement warrants the extended use of the medication that seems most effective.

If the child exhibits agitation or if there is no observable change with the drug, the medication will not be helpful. If extreme quietness is noted with the drug, it suggests that a smaller dose would be more beneficial.

To avoid the embarrassment of taking pills in school, the single-dose Dexedrine Spansule in a 5- or 10-mg dose or the Benzedrine Spansule in a 15-mg dose is preferred. It is prescribed after breakfast. The effect will start within an hour and last until mid-afternoon. Occasionally it may be necessary to prescribe a half or whole tablet of specific amphetamine for after-school hyperactivity.

A single 20-mg dose of methylphenidate can be prescribed at breakfast. It is less effective than the twice-a-day dosage; however, a prolonged action form is almost ready for approval and it seems as effective as the amphetamine spansule form.

Pemoline magnesium (Cylert) is a new long-acting central nervous system stimulant. While it is structurally dissimilar from the

TABLE 5
Attention Span Rating by Time Samples

MEDICATION					ACTIVITIES			BEHAVIOR	REMARKS
NAME	DATE	HOUR	MG	FORM T,S,E	TASK STANDARDIZED	TIME ON TASK - + ++ +++	RATING I NC W	EXCESSIVE X,N,D,H,T,O	
NONE d-AMPHETAMINE METHYLPHENIDATE d-ℓ AMPHETAMINE OTHERS					MOTOR READING COPYING ARITHMETIC OTHERS				

CODE –

RATING
- I = IMPROVED
- NC = NO CHANGE
- W = WORSE

MEDICATION
- T = TABLET
- S = SPANSULE
- E = ELIXER

TIME ON TASK
- – UNDER 5 sec.
- + 5—9 sec.
- ++ 10—14 sec.
- +++ 14 OR MORE

EXCESSIVE BEHAVIOR
- X = MOVEMENT
- N = NOISES
- D = DISTURBANCES
- H = HEADTURNING
- T = TALKING
- O = OTHERS

amphetamines or methylphenidate, it has a similar action. It is administered as a single oral dose each morning in a range of from 18.75 to 112.5 mg, with an average dose of 75 mg a day.

While pemoline cannot yet be assessed for its long-term benefits, dose for dose it does not appear to be more effective than either amphetamines or methylphenidate. It takes between 3 and 4 weeks to observe a beneficial effect on attention span. Its major attraction is the single morning dose schedule and its availability as a nonrestricted prescription item. Table 6 provides information about dosage and schedules of administering these medications.[6]

Adverse Effects. Common complaints associated with the amphetamines are poor appetite, weight loss, difficulty in going to sleep or restless patterns of sleep, dark circles under the eyes with facial pallor, and vague abdominal complaints. Caloric intake may be reduced substantially. There are much fewer complaints with methylphenidate.

With pemoline, sleeplessness occurs in 30% of poor responders and 9% of good responders.

Summer drug holidays, small doses, and concentrated caloric foods can help neutralize the effects of undernutrition or growth deprivation.

We have failed to confirm linear growth deprivation with Dexedrine. In 48 children receiving 10-mg Dexedrine Spansule for 12 months, with medication holidays during long vacations, there were no significant changes in height before, during, or after drug administration. It is likely that such drugs used continuously in large doses over long periods have a potential to produce growth deprivation.

Alternative Approaches

There is a high degree of parent and public resistance to the use of psychostimulant medication. Alternate approaches are available but the effects are as yet unclear.

Food Additives. Food allergy or sensitivity to additives in food can produce a "tension-fatigue" syndrome, which has been declared a cause of hyperactivity.[7] It is logical to conclude that irritability resulting from food intolerance can produce fidgeting, which can stimulate hyperkinesis. The results are inconclusive in controlled studies of subjects on additive-free diets.[8]

Caffeine. Coffee and caffeine have been recommended as alternatives to psychostimulants to control hyperkinesis. A double-blind study, however, showed that 10 mg/day of methylphenidate was significantly more effective than 160 mg/day of caffeine.[9]

TABLE 6
Medications to Improve Attention Span

MEDICATION	mg/kg	mg/day	METHOD OF PRESCRIBING
d-AMPHETAMINE (DEXEDRINE SULFATE)	0.25–1.0	2.5–40	1 TABLET 8 AM + NOON; ? ½–1 TABLET AT 3PM 1 SPANSULE 8 AM; ? ½–1 TABLET AT 3PM
d-ℓ AMPHETAMINE (BENZIDRINE SULFATE)	0.5–2.0	5.0–80	1 TABLET 8 AM + NOON; ? ½–1 TABLET AT 3PM 1 SPANSULE 8 AM; ? ½–1 TABLET AT 3PM
METHYLPHENIDATE (RITALIN)	0.25–2.0	5.0–80	1 TABLET 8 AM + NOON; ?-1 TABLET AT 3PM DOUBLE DOSE PRN.
PEMOLINE (CYLERT)	1.9–2.6	17.5–112.50	1–2 TABLETS AT BREAKFAST

Hypoglycemia. Some children who are unable to respond to stress have flat or inconsistent (high-low) 5-hour glucose tolerance curves. Such children may be hyperactive. A gluten-free diet and/or the elimination of dextrose or crude sugars has been recommended to improve behavior. Except in true cases of hypoglycemia or malabsorption syndrome, proof is lacking that there is a relationship between inconsistent glucose values, low-sugar, gluten-free diets and hyperkinesis.

Megavitamins. Excessively large doses of nicotine acid, pyridoxine, ascorbic acid, and pantothenic acid are purported to alleviate hyperkinesis. They have not been studied in a controlled fashion.[10]

Behavior Modification. Behavioral interventions, both positive and negative reinforcement, operant conditioning, and self-controlled training are being used to replace psychostimulant medication. The effectiveness of these methods is still unproven because of insufficient controlled studies. Yet these methods do appear effective in cases of undifferentiated hyperactivity.[11] However, children with true hyperkinetic impulse disorder often respond poorly to behavior modification when it is used without medication.[12] Wender postulates that it is because both pleasure and pain responses are impaired as a result of hypothalamic dysfunction.[13]

Discussion

A point of contention in recent years concerns whether there is a clear relationship between adverse perinatal events and later outcome in mildly involved children. Minkowski and co-workers confirmed the studies of 7-year outcome reported here.[14] Their research suggests that persisting symptoms which reflect neurologic dysfunctions are better indicators of future problems than the actual causes. They discuss the role of intrauterine asphyxia in the development of late sequelae. The evidence supports an unclear relationship and suggests that stable environment, good nutrition, and enrichment can compensate for early stress. Whether MBD represents a stage in development during which the central nervous system is being adapted to environmental needs cannot yet be answered.

Another point recently confirmed by Denckla and Rudel is of great importance to the clinician. On controlled studies there were significant differences in involuntary and overflow movements (associated movements) as well as differences in dysrhythmia found in children performing repetitive heel-toe, toe-tapping, or repetitive finger tasks. These involuntary movements can be noted by watching the child's hands when the fingers are outstretched. Associated movements are observed when an involuntary repetitive movement occurs in one hand when it is being performed by the other (example, with both hands outstretched, but fingers closed, when the fingers of the left hand are abducted voluntarily, similar movement occurs in the right hand). Denckla and Rudel conclude that these associated (overflow) movements appear to be the stigmata of deficient motor inhibition/control and are central to identifying the hyperkinetic-MBD syndrome.[15]

Summary

1. MBD of perinatal origin is easiest to identify by history and neurologic findings and responds best to psychostimulant medication.

2. Objective rating scales are helpful in evaluating drug responses.

3. Psychostimulant medication, when used in conjunction with other appropriate supportive measures, is of documented value in the management of MBD.

4. Some alternative methods are worthy of trial, but clear proof of their value is lacking.

References

1. Denhoff, E., and Tarnopol, L.: Medical responsibilities in learning disorders. In *Learning Disorders in Children: Diagnosis, Medication, Education*, L. Tarnopol, Ed. Little, Brown, Boston, 1971, pp. 65–118.
2. Niswander, K.R., and Gordon, M.: *The Women and Their Pregnancies.* W.B. Saunders, Philadelphia, 1972.
3. Safer, D.J., and Allen, R.P.: *Hyperactive Children.* University Park Press, Baltimore, 1976, p. 16.
4. Denhoff, E., Hainsworth, P.K., and Hainsworth, M.: The child at risk for learning disorder. Can he be identified during the first year of life? *Clin Pediatr* **2:** 164, 1972.
5. Schain, R.J.: *Neurology of Childhood Learning Disorders.* Williams & Wilkins, Baltimore, 1972, pp. 9–28.
6. Denhoff, E.: Minimal brain dysfunction and stimulant drugs: Indications, dosage and side effects. *Hosp Form* **2:** 328, 1976.
7. Campbell, M.B.: Tension-fatigue syndrome. *Otolaryngol Clin North Am* **7:** 805, 1971.
8. Kolata, G.B.: Childhood hyperactivity: A new look at treatment and causes. *Science* **199:** 515, 1978.
9. Garfinkle, B.D., Webster, C.D., and Solomons, L.: Methylphenidate and caffeine in the treatment of hyperkinetic children. *Am J Psychiatry* **132:** 7, 1975.
10. Statement, Committee on Nutrition, American Academy of Pediatrics. Megavitamin therapy for childhood psychosis and learning disabilities. *Pediatrics* **5:** 910, 1976.
11. Stewart, M., and Olds, S.W.: *Raising a Hyperactive Child.* Harper & Row, New York, 1973, pp. 127–188.
12. Benesche, H.I.: Performance of Hyperkinetic and Normal Children under

two conditions of reinforcement. Thesis, Department of Psychology, University of Rhode Island, 1974.
13. Wender, P.H.: *Minimal Brain Dysfunction in Children.* Wiley/Interscience, New York, 1971.
14. Minkowski, A., Amiel-Tison, C., Cukier, F., Dreyfus-Brisac, C., Reher, J.P., and de Bethman, O.: Long term follow-up and sequelae of asphyxiated infants. In *Intrauterine Asphyxia and the Developing Fetal Brain,* L. Gluck, Ed. Yearbook Medical Publishers, Chicago, 1977, pp. 309–330.
15. Denckla, M.B., and Rudel, R.G.: Anomalies of motor development in hyperactive boys. *Ann Neurol* **3:** 231, 1978.

5

Neurophysiologic and Biochemical Aspects of Hyperkinesis

Taranath Shetty, M.D.

Probably the earliest observation of a neurophysiologic abnormality in the hyperkinetic syndrome was the description by Werner and Strauss[1] of the difficulty these children had in differentiating a figure from its background. Laufer, Denhoff, and Solomons[2] then demonstrated yet another neurophysiologic alteration with the use of the photometrazol test and also showed that the lower threshold to photometrazol activation in hyperkinetic children can be altered toward normality with the use of amphetamines. They postulated that amphetamines probably had an effect on the inhibitory portion of the reticular activating system. Another neurophysiologic difference from normal subjects, pointed out in their original paper, is the paradoxical response to phenobarbitol therapy.

Since hyperkinesis consists of several subgroups which result in the same clinical syndrome through similar effects on common neuronal and biochemical pathways, the electrophysiologic and biochemical alterations recognized in some patients with this syndrome might well be epiphenomena rather than causally related.

Clinical Assistant Professor of Pediatrics, Brown University Medical Program, Section of Reproductive and Developmental Medicine, Brown University, Providence, Rhode Island.

The major support for the organic versus emotional basis of this syndrome comes from the compelling evidence that appropriate doses of amphetamines or related analeptics can, at least in part, alleviate most motor and behavioral abnormalities attending this syndrome.

In the past, much has been written on the neurophysiologic and biochemical alterations from normal in this syndrome. Some of the data are confusing and controversial. For this reason we undertook studies of our own. The work began with a systematic study of EEGs in these children at the Neurophysiology Department of Children's Hospital in Boston. It was very soon evident that a large majority of these children had a poorly maintained EEG background with very little well-sustained alpha activity. Follow-up studies of EEGs showed that, with increasing age and decreasing hyperkinesis, alpha activity increased in amount and organization.[3]

The next step was to determine the effects of short-term administration of amphetamines on the amount of alpha activity and to compare the resulting changes in behavior and performance on long-term therapy.

The beneficial effects of intravenous amphetamines in a dose of 10 mg/m^2 in a child who showed very poor alpha activity in the predrug EEG was dramatic (Fig. 1).

The same phenomenon was produced with an injection of 20 mg/m^2 of intravenous methylphenidate in another hyperkinetic child.

These results led to a study using equal volumes of IV amphetamine, methylphenidate, and saline in random order in a double-blind test involving 28 children and 5 controls. The EEG responses were collected on magnetic tape 15 minutes before and 15 minutes after the injection and subjected to a Fourier transformation, using a PDP-12 computer. The results showed an increase in alpha activity in those children who responded to therapy on a long-term basis but not on those who did not. Coincidentally, all control subjects also showed a consistent increase in alpha activity on stimulant injection. Since alpha rhythm in the human EEG is an index of relaxed wakefulness and habituation to a class of stimuli results in augmentation of alpha, if alpha rhythms can be considered a measure of attention span, our results support the hypothesis that the basic neurophysiologic defect in hyperkinesis of childhood is a disorder of inhibitory mechanisms in the brain. Irrelevant stimuli are not filtered out and the child is at the mercy of all the stimuli in his environment. Our study indicates that CNS stimulant drugs act by strengthening these inhibitory mechanisms.[4]

A by-product of the study was an opportunity to confirm indi-

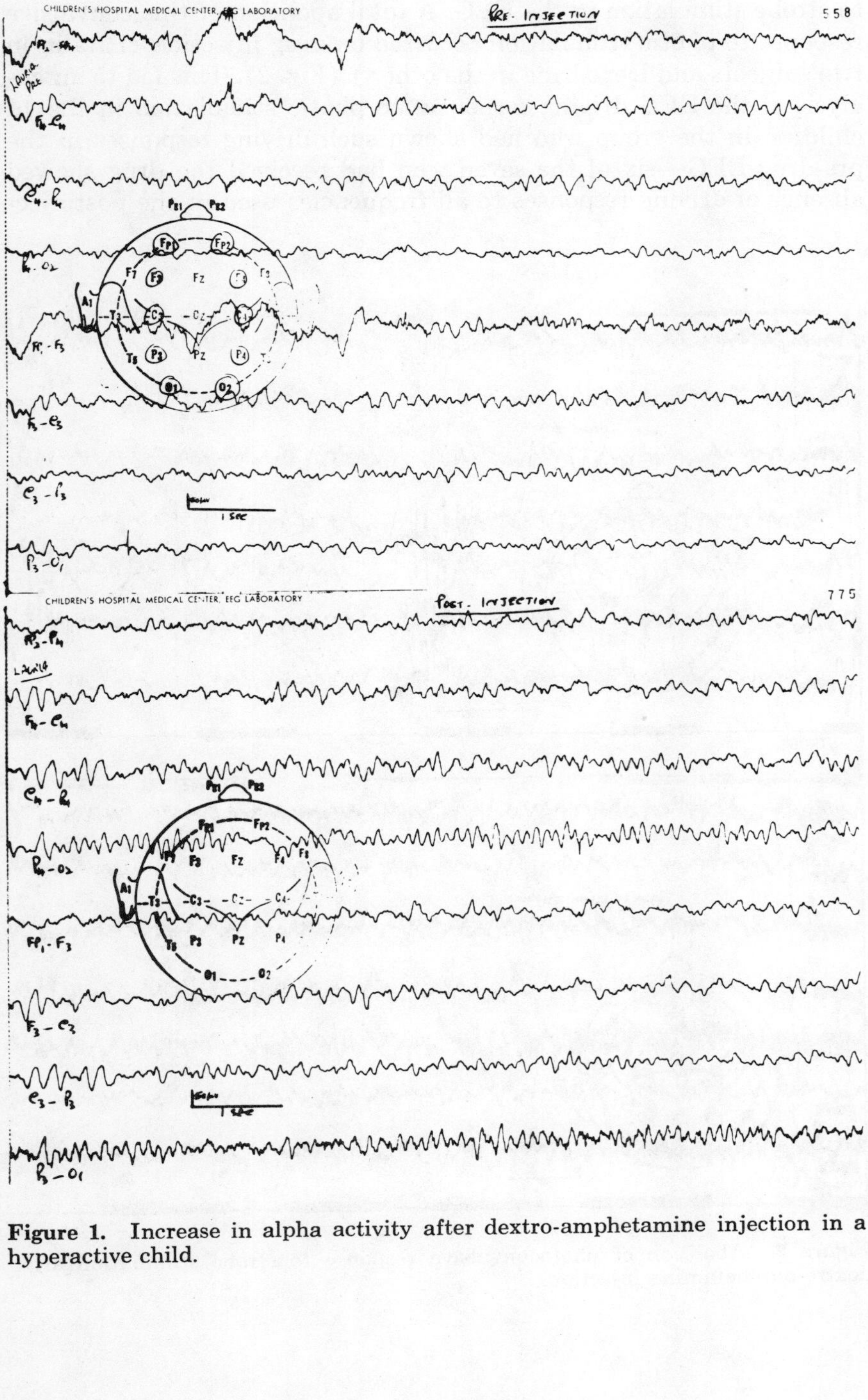

Figure 1. Increase in alpha activity after dextro-amphetamine injection in a hyperactive child.

rectly the unreplicated photometrazol study of Laufer and associates. There were three children in the study with photoconvulsive responses to strobe stimulation in the EEG. A total abolition of this convulsive response to photic stimulation occurred on drug injection (Ritalin in two subjects and Dexedrine in the other.) (Fig. 2). This led to an analysis of the EEG driving responses to photic stimulation in the 11 children in the group who had shown such driving responses in the pre-drug EEG—six of the seven who had received the drug showed absence of driving responses to all frequencies used in the postinjec-

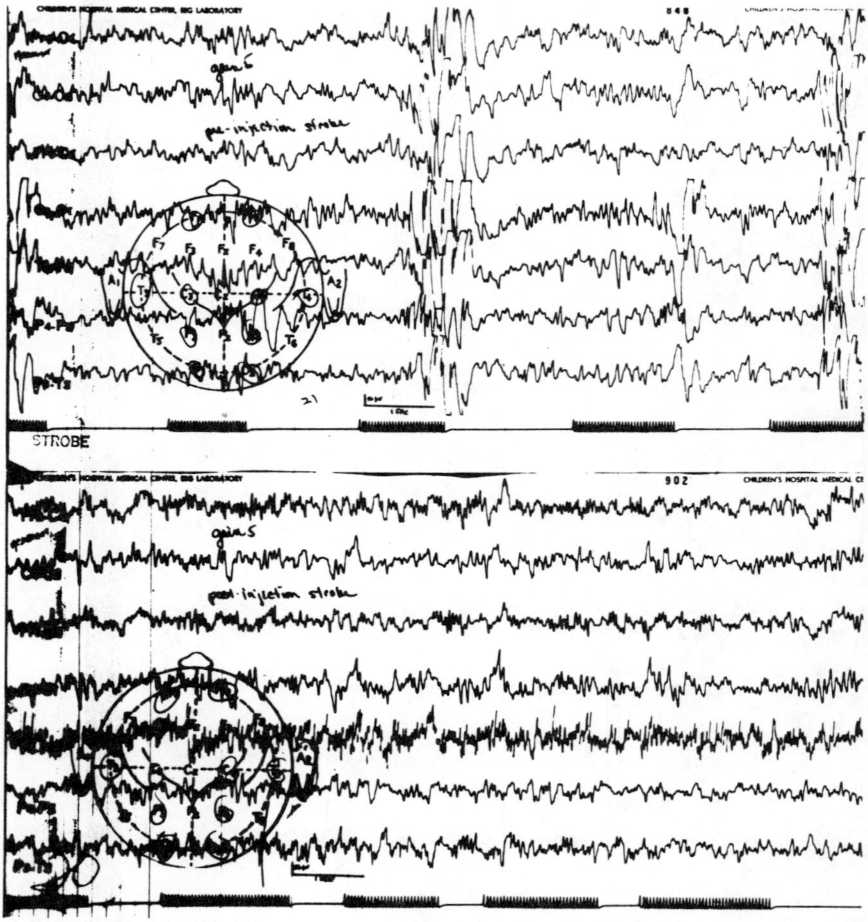

Figure 2. Abolition of photoconvulsive response to strobe stimulation after dextro-amphetamine injection.

tion period. Four children who received saline and the controls showed no alteration of their driving responses. These results again suggested a neurophysiologic difference from normal individuals. Enhancement of the central adrenergic state is known to decrease driving responses to photic stimulation, and our results seemed to indicate indirectly that stimulant drugs are able to enhance central adrenergic mechanisms to a greater degree in hyperactive children as compared with normal ones.[5]

Since amphetamines are well known to influence central catecholamine mediated neural function, the next logical step was the direct measurement of metabolites of catecholamines and indoleamines in the spinal fluid of hyperkinetic children and the study of their alteration, if any, by amphetamines. To our disappointment, CFS levels of homovanillic acid (HVA) and 5-hydroxy-indolacetic acid (5 HIAA), the principal metabolites of dopamine and serotonin, were not significantly different from those of age-matched controls.[6] However, it should be added that we measured only steady-state levels, and a better way to measure the synthesis and release of the parent amine in the central nervous system is to employ the probenecid technique

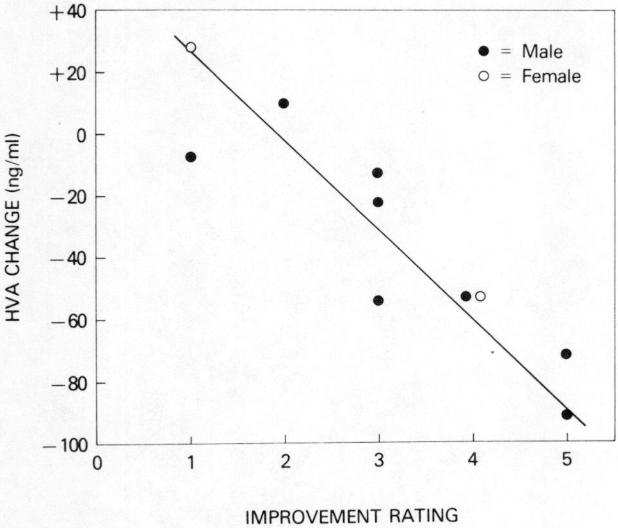

Figure 3. Relation between dextro-amphetamine-induced change in CSF HVA levels and clinical improvement.

to block the efflux of these metabolites from the CSFX. Using the latter method, Shaywitz[7] has recently reported a significant difference in HVA levels in six hyperkinetic children.

However, we did demonstrate that at dose levels that suppress hyperkinetic behavior in children, amphetamines did decrease spinal fluid HVA values and that there was a correlation between the degree of clinical improvement and HVA reduction (Fig. 3). These results support the hypothesis that dopaminergic mechanisms contribute to the pathogenesis of childhood hyperkinesis and that the efficacy of stimulant drugs in part reflects a disease-related alteration in central neurohormonal mechanisms.

References

1. Werner, H., and Strauss, A.: Pathology of figure ground relation in the child. *J Abnorm Soc Psychol* **36:** 58, 1941.
2. Laufer, M.W., Denhoff, E., and Solomons, G.: Hyperkinetic impulse disorder in children's behavior problems. *Psychosom Med* **19:** 38, 1957.
3. Shetty, T.: Alpha rhythms and hyperkinesis. *Nature* **241:** 563, 1973.
4. Shetty, T.: Alpha rhythms in the hyperkinetic child. *Nature* **234:** 476, 1971.
5. Shetty, T.: Photic responses in hyperkinesis of childhood. *Science* **174:** 1356–1357, 1971.
6. Shetty, T., and Chase, T.N.: Central monoamines and hyperkinesis of childhood. *Neurology* **26:** 1000–1002, 1976.
7. Shaywitz, B.A., Cohen, D.J., and Bower, M.B.: CSF monoamine metabolites in children with minimal brain dysfunction: Evidence for alteration of brain dopamine. *J Pediat* **90:** 67–71, 1977.

6

Learning Curves of Hyperkinetic Children—The Habituation Response

Allan Berman, Ph.D.

Many observers have noted that hyperkinetic children have difficulties in most standard classroom situations. They are usually described as distractible, inattentive, unable to concentrate, and the like. Very frequently it is the learning inefficiency of the hyperkinetic child which first brings the parent or teacher to the professional seeking some type of help. Reitan[3] has found that, of those children considered hyperkinetic, or minimally brain damaged, the presenting symptoms are as likely to be academic as behavioral in nature. Others have also found that hyperkinetic children present unique difficulties for the educator, whether or not the child is presenting other behavioral problems.

Since many hyperkinetic children are successfully treated with medication, it is not surprising that observers have found that those children being successfully treated with medication also show more typical learning patterns; that is, medication seems to "normalize" the youngsters, both in and out of the classroom. The purpose of this chapter is not to speculate on the problems of defining hyperkinesis, nor is it to pass judgment on the effectiveness of treatment with medication. The purpose is rather to look more closely at three

University of Rhode Island, Kingston, Rhode Island.

recent studies done in our department. These studies were all done for the purpose of studying some problem of hyperkinetic children and, as part of their design, all used comparisons between hyperkinetics, on and off medication, and normals on various learning tasks. The studies were done independently and for different reasons, but close scrutiny of their results suggests that the three, taken together, may yield important information about exactly what aspect of the learning situation is most affected by hyperkinesis, as well as by subsequent medication.

The three studies all were done at the University of Rhode Island Psychology Department, where we have been attempting to understand the effect of hyperkinesis on psychological processes, and the effect on these processes of the medications used in treatment of hyperkinesis.

The first study was done by Thomas Walsh.[4] His main purpose was to investigate Wender's anhedonia hypothesis, that hyperkinetic children would be less responsive to both positive and negative reinforcers of behavior. The design was carefully constructed to compare three groups of children: hyperkinetics receiving medication, hyperkinetics not receiving medication, and normals. The pertinent aspect of this study is the part that investigated the effect of negative reinforcement on the learning of a simple motor task, and the frequency of the learned response. The subjects had to squeeze a rubber hand pump to displace water from one container to another. While doing so, they wore a standard blood pressure cuff which was inflated so as to cause ischemic muscle pain after a short time. Subjects were asked to pump until they felt pain, whereupon the cuff was removed, and the amount of water displaced was recorded as the dependent variable. Three trial periods were used to determine whether, over time, the subjects in the different groups became more or less able to pump water, knowing that the pain would occur.

Walsh found, among other things, that hyperkinetics receiving medication performed more like normals than did hyperkinetics not receiving medication. In this case, hyperkinetics on medication and normals showed a gradual increase in the amount of water pumped over the three trial periods, while hyperkinetics not on medication showed a significant decrease in amount pumped.

While these findings were not very supportive of the anhedonia hypothesis, some additional information, not related to the hypotheses under study, was interesting. The results were expressed in mean amounts of water displaced over the three trial periods. Studying the graphs of individual trial responses, it seemed obvious that most of the variability among groups occurred during the first trial period, while nearly no variability was detectable during later trials.

To test this notion, the data for the latter two trials were recomputed separately from those for the first trial. This recalculation showed more definitively that nearly all the differences between groups occurred during the first trial.

By itself, that finding was not as suggestive as it became after another study by Howard Benesch.[1] The purpose of this study was to determine how primary versus social reinforcers differentially effect the performance of hyperkinetic children. Once again, three groups were used. This time the task was to drop a golf ball through a hole. Subjects received either primary (food) or social reinforcers, and the dependent variable was the number of balls dropped in a given period. Once again, differences were found between reinforcers as well as among groups, and when results for the first group of trials were separated from those for later trials, it was demonstrated that nearly all of the variability occurred in the early trials.

We are involved in another study, this time attempting to determine the effect of medication on the hyperkinetic's ability to learn simple verbal paired-associate tasks, with a hypothesis regarding the effect of hyperkinesis on auditory memory skills. Again we have three groups: hyperkinetic on medication, hyperkinetic off medication, and normal. Again there are several trials under different conditions of reinforcement. Our original design had been to do the study much as others have keen done, that is, to determine the mean response over the trial period. However, this time we have the knowledge of the previous two studies and are also calculating the results and differences among groups for each separate trial period. We are finding astonishingly similar findings to those mentioned previously. Although it was not the purpose of our paired-associate study, we are again finding that most of the variability among groups can be accounted for by the first stages of learning—the earliest trials. Later trials provide very few differences among groups.

What stands out, then, are the three similar but serendipitous findings in three independent studies designed to study different hypotheses, using different tasks and different subjects. Yet on all three—one simple motor task, one task involving a visual/motor response, and another task involving the learning of auditorily presented verbal material—it appeared that, while hyperkinetics receiving medication perform more like normals than non-medicated hyperkinetics, nearly all differences in performance can be accounted for by differences occurring during the earliest phase of learning.

As we have tried to understand the meaning of this information, an explanation that seems obvious to start with is that, if differences in learning occur primarily during the earliest phase of learning, then the learning problems of hyperkinetic children may not be gross learning difficulties at all, but rather some type of dysfunction in the habituation phenomenon. The more we explore this idea, the more intriguing it becomes as an explanation not only for the learning difficulties hyperkinetics encounter but also for other aspects of their behavior.

Briefly put, habituation refers to the very first stage of learning. Experimental psychologists have known for some time that, in animals, habituation is a phenomenon that occurs predictably and is one that must be accounted for during research on animal learning. Animals must be given an opportunity to become familiar with the environment prior to the commencement of a learning task, or else ensuing learning curves will be inaccurate. Most schools do not have to be concerned about habituation because most children adapt to the learning situation quickly, and the habituation transfers readily from one learning situation to another.

Yet, if habituation is the problem for hyperkinetics, as the studies above seem to suggest, then these assumptions about the rapidity and fluidity of human habituation may not be accurate for hyperkinetic children. A logical conclusion from the incidental data presented from the three studies is that hyperkinetic children require a longer habituation time than do nonhyperkinetics, and that habituation in hyperkinetics does not transfer as readily from one situation to another. In practical terms, these conclusions mean that hyperkinetics need longer exposure to new learning situations before they are required to learn anything, simply to become accustomed to functioning in the learning situation. Furthermore, hyperkinetics seem to have difficulty transferring this habituation from one situation to another. So that, while we have become accustomed to the fact that many children can readily adapt, for example, from one classroom to another, or from one subject area to another, hyperkinetics apparently require longer to make the change.

Examining these conclusions, with respect to what we can observe clinically about hyperkinetics, the observations and the conclusions from the data seem appropriate. Hyperkinetic children are frequently described as unable to settle down, or distractible, or unable to concentrate. These reactions may be due simply to the fact that, in school, most children are moved fairly often and fairly quickly through different learning situations. Indeed, some new teaching strategies promote frequent changes in learning situations to help combat boredom. While these approaches may be appropriate for normal children, the data reviewed here suggest that the approaches are not at all appropriate, and may even further penalize the hyperkinetic child who may be having great difficulty shifting from one learning situation to another.

These suggestions must, of course, be studied more closely before any firm action can be recommended. The present conclusions are drawn from results of three separate studies, none of which was intended to study habituation. But the phenomenon of habituation is well known to experimental psychologists, and methods of studying its effects and parameters are available. What is not so readily available are appropriate methods for use with human subjects, as well as tasks which provide for some generalizability. Therefore, the first recommendation for future action must be for researchers to begin to study more closely the phenomenon of habituation in children, more specifically whether or not habituation curves differ between hyperkinetics and nonhyperkinetics. Experience suggests that any differences may be interrelated with age variables, so these studies will have to control carefully for age level in the groups involved.

Dr. Sol Gordon[2] has said that "there is no reason why knowledge gained in one field of study cannot be used by individuals in other fields of study." People who have been studying the learning problems of hyperkinetic children have most frequently not been utilizing some of the basic techniques and principles developed in experimental psychology for the study of learning processes. The fact that habituation, an elementary concept, has not been systematically studied in children with learning problems suggests that perhaps it would be useful for those who study learning problems as they appear clinically to organize their research around the learning paradigms found so effective in the experimental laboratories. This has been done to some degree in the study of infant learning, but not in the study of older children who experience learning problems. Thus, not only is habituation important for more detailed research, but so are the other known phases of the learning process.

Aside from suggesting further research that must be done, the present analysis also suggests several other types of activities that could be undertaken. All of the studies referred to used three groups: a control group of normals, along with medicated and nonmedicated groups of hyperkinetics. The results of all of the studies suggested that medicated hyperkinetics perform more like normals, and it is the nonmedicated hyperkinetics whose performance is discrepant. If this can indeed be generalized, we might also conclude that the most significant effect of medication on learning in hyperkinetic children is to normalize the children's habituation curve, that is, to enable the hyperkinetic to habituate to new situations more quickly and to concentrate faster. These conclusions also suggest that *medication might not play nearly so important a role in effecting learning after the habituation period.*

Aside from suggesting even more research possibilities, this last conclusion also has important implications for clinical practice for both physicians and educators. If hyperkinetics need more habituation time and less frequent changes in learning situations, and if medication reduces these needs, the educational and curriculum planner for the child and the physician in charge of treatment might be able to collaborate for the most effective use of medication during habituation, while reducing the use of medication during other phases of learning. Perhaps judicious use of educational planning would minimize new or changing learning situations enough so that minimal use of medication would be needed.

Conclusion

Studies intended for research into other aspects of hyperkinesis have produced incidental data suggesting that habituation may be a key element in understanding the learning problems of hyperkinetics. These suggestions are based on the assumption that these conclusions from the incidenttal data of three studies are indeed correct.

Since we still know relatively little about the mechanisms of hyperkinesis and minimal brain dysfunction and how they effect the learning processes, it is not unrealistic to agree that we might not always wait for experimental proof of our hypotheses before taking some type of remediative clinical action. Thus, while hoping that those who deal with the education and treatment of these children will incorporate these suggestions into their treatment strategies, we would also hope that these suggestions will stimulate further clinical research that needs to be done in this area if we are to be able to understand and plan for these youngsters more efficiently.

References

1. Benesch, H.: Performance of hyperkinetic and normal children under two conditions of reinforcement. Doctoral dissertation, University of Rhode Island, 1975.
2. Gordon, S.: Personal communication, 1974.
3. Reitan, R.: Neuropsychological studies of minimal brain damage in children. (In press, 1975.)
4. Walsh, T.: Anhedonia as a symptom of minimal brain dysfunction in children. Doctoral dissertation, University of Rhode Island, 1975.

The cited doctoral dissertations, done at the University of Rhode Island, were the basis for some of the conclusions referred to in this paper. Copies may be obtained through the *Dissertation Abstracts* available at most libraries, or by writing to the author.

7

Laboratory Measurement of Hyperactive Children's Response to Stimulant Medication

Marcel Kinsbourne, M.D., James Swanson, Ph.D., and
Dorothy Herman, B.Sc.

Stimulants have been used extensively for the clinical treatment of chronically inattentive, distractible, and impulsive ("hyperactive") children for 35 years, beginning with Bradley's work[1] reported in 1937. No attempt will be made to review the literature on this topic, since comprehensive reviews exist.[2–6] Nor will the arguments for[2] and against[7] the use of this treatment be repeated here. Instead, we will present data from our research program, which was designed to answer a neutral and fundamental question: What is the immediate behavioral effect of a single therapeutic dose of stimulant medication on children with symptoms of hyperactivity? Specifically, information will be presented concerning the effect of an acute administration of methylphenidate (Ritalin) on cognitive functioning, based on objective measurement of behavior under the controlled conditions of the laboratory. The diagnostic usefulness of this information for evaluation of the hyperkinetic impulse disorder in children will be discussed.

Neuropsychology Research Unit, The Hospital for Sick Children, Toronto, Ontario, Canada.

The Diagnostic Drug Trial

Not all children who manifest symptoms of hyperactivity respond favorably to stimulants. Bradley[9] noted this in his initial study of hyperactive children in a group home, and more recent investigations have confirmed his findings. Regardless of which stimulant is used, less than 70% of those children identified by history as being hyperactive actually respond favorably to stimulant therapy.[10] Twenty years ago, Laufer and Denhoff[11] formally proposed an operational definition of hyperactivity based on response to stimulant drugs. They recommended that a *diagnostic drug trial* be given to children with symptoms of the hyperkinetic impulse disorder, and that "a favorable response to amphetamine is supportive evidence for a diagnosis of the hyperkinetic syndrome." The clinical utility of this approach has been proven over the years, and the use of the diagnostic drug trial continues to be recommended by many investigators in this area, including Wender,[2] Safer and Allen,[4] Cantwell,[3] and Kinsbourne.[6]

Presumably, if a favorable response to stimulant therapy is taken as supportive evidence *for* the hyperkinetic syndrome, then an adverse response to stimulant therapy should be taken as evidence *against* the hyperkinetic syndrome. Since only about two-thirds of all children identified by history as being hyperactive actually respond favorably to stimulant therapy, one must carefully assess the response to a trial on stimulants to ensure that the significant minority of hyperactive children (the adverse responders) is not incorrectly treated with stimulant drugs.

Evaluating Response to Stimulants

How does one determine if stimulants work when they are tried? Solomons[12] and Safer and Allen[4] give detailed descriptions of how drug trials can be evaluated by the pediatrician. Small doses should be tried initially, and increases should be made if no improvement is noted. Over an extended period following this kind of stepwise increase in stimulant dosage, one of two outcomes will occur: at some level of medication, either an obvious improvement in behavior will result (a favorable response), or a "toxic" effect on behavior will result (an adverse response). If the adverse response occurs at the initial dose, or a favorable response does not occur before an adverse response emerges, then the child can be classified as an "adverse responder." If a favorable response emerges before an adverse response occurs, then the adverse response can be interpreted as an overdose effect, and the child can be classified as a favorable responder at a lower dose. Solomons[12] has suggested that telephone contact with parents over a 2-month period is sufficient for monitoring a child's response to a diagnostic drug trial, and that this method can be used to determine the optimum level of medication for an individual patient. Others think that parent and teacher questionnaires are a more objective and desirable means of eliciting subjective impressions of a child's response to medication.

Conners[13,14] developed parent and teacher questionnaires which are now widely used. By having a parent or teacher rate a child on critical dimensions of behavior related to hyperactivity, one can obtain an overall *hyperactivity index* for that particular child. A valuable feature of Conners's rating scale is that norms are available and can be used to determine the degree of a child's hyperactivity. A score of over 15 on the hyperactivity index is two standard deviations above the norm.

Schain and Reynard,[15] among others, have noted that subjective ratings of drug effects have many limitations. More objective measures of drug response, not dependent on the tolerance of observers, may be derived from performance on tasks in a laboratory setting.

Laboratory Evaluation of Response

Many laboratory studies have been conducted to investigate the response of hyperactive children to medication, but few have emphasized the difference between favorable and adverse responders to stimulants. The emphasis, instead, has been on the response of the group of favorable responders, with some emphasis on different types or patterns of the favorable response to stimulant therapy. One of the most comprehensive studies of this type was reported by Conners,[16] who included in his study less than two-thirds of the patients initially referred with symptoms suggesting hyperactivity. Conners used a variety of drug–placebo difference scores derived from questionnaires and laboratory tests to determine the pattern of drug response in a large group of favorable responders.

However, a crucial aspect of diagnosing hyperactivity is the identification of those children who will *not* react favorably, or the adverse responders. The 1971 HEW Conference[17] emphasized this, as have several others. Grinspoon and his co-workers have concluded that "there has been no way of predicting beforehand which students will profit from which, if any, drugs" (Grinspoon and Hedbloom,[7] p. 254), and that "the possible adverse effects of these (stimulant) drugs" requires a more careful approach to prescribing them.[18]

How does one adopt a more careful approach to prescribing stimulant drugs, if the adverse responders cannot be identified on the basis of history? The type of diagnostic drug trial proposed by Laufer and Denhoff[11] and endorsed by many others is one way, but it is lengthy and relies on untrained observers whose subjective criteria are undefined. Schmitt[8] has labeled the diagnostic trial as the greatest misuse of stimulant drugs because it exposes many more children to these drugs than are likely to benefit from them.

Objective measurement of the initial response of a child with symptoms of hyperactivity to an acute administration of stimulant medication (rather than relying on the subjective assessment of behavior changes associated with prolonged use of stimulants), is a diagnostic technique that may be useful. It identifies the adverse responder quickly so as to prevent mistreatment with drugs. If this refinement of the diagnostic trial proves to be successful, it would satisfy some legitimate concerns of critics of the current practice of prescribing stimulant drugs to diagnose hyperactivity.

Revision of the Diagnostic Drug Trial

Kinsbourne[19] has suggested that initial (acute) response to stimulant medication is comparable in direction and extent to the long-term effect reported in the literature, and thus introduced a diagnostic drug trial based on a single dose of medication. Using the short-acting stimulant methylphenidate (Ritalin), Kinsbourne[19] established drug and placebo conditions within an individual across only 2 days of testing and obtained results similar to the usual double-blind crossover experiments comparing behavior in drug and placebo treatment conditions extending over periods of weeks. In addition to a questionnaire (the Junior Eysenck Personality Inventory), performances on the Porteus Mazes and Critical Flicker Fusion frequency were measured. All three measures produced statistically significant differences between drug and placebo conditions.

Swanson and Kinsbourne[20] refined this method to establish drug and placebo states within a single day for each individual. They also introduced the paired-associate learning test for laboratory monitoring of both the adverse and the favorable effects of medication on cognitive functioning. Using the same learning task to monitor drug responsiveness, Kinsbourne, Roberts, and Swanson[21] reported data obtained in 2 days of laboratory testing which is consistent with data obtained from traditional long-term diagnostic drug trials. They found that, of 75 consecutive children referred to the Learning Clinic of the Hospital for Sick Children with a complaint of hyperactive behavior, only 53 responded favorably to stimulant medication, and thus replicated the work of Bradley[9] and Fish.[22] Those favorable responders, as a group, showed drug-related improvement in the learning task performed in the laboratory, while the remaining 30% (labeled adverse responders), as a group, showed significant drug-related impairment on the same task. Their suggestion was that response to acute administration of stimulant drug is the same in direction and extent as response to long-term use, and thus the acute response could be used to diagnose favorable and adverse responders to stimulant therapy.

The purpose of the present paper is to describe the 2-day, double-blind procedure that we have used as an acute diagnostic drug trial in the laboratory. In addition to the description of our procedures, we will present data from our research program and will discuss the practical and theoretical usefulness of this paradigm.

The Acute (2-Day) Drug–Placebo Trial

Methylphenidate, the stimulant drug most often prescribed for hyperactive children, has a restricted active life: When taken orally, its action starts in 30 minutes and its effective duration is about 4 hours. These properties allow an investigator to establish a drug state and a non drug (placebo) state within an individual in a single day. Our procedure is based on behavior differences observed in the laboratory when drug and placebo states are established in this way in a double-blind fashion. Immediate changes in behavior associated with drug and placebo states occur, allowing us to determine objectively, in a short period, which children respond favorably and which adversely to stimulant medication. The schedule, developed for investigating stimulant-related state-dependent learning, but now extended to include several tests, is described below:

8:30 A.M.	Medication (drug or placebo)
9:00 A.M.	Breakfast
9:30 A.M.–11:30 A.M.	Testing
12:30 P.M.	Medication (opposite state established)
1:00 P.M.	Lunch
1:30 P.M.–3:30 P.M.	Testing

Several special features of our paradigm must be noted. First, each patient is tested on 2 successive days using the same schedule, but performance on the first day is considered as practice and is ignored. Second, medication (usually methylphenidate) is given 30 minutes before meals to minimize (or hold constant) the effect of the digestive processes on the absorption of the medication. Yoss and Daly[23] have indicated that methylphenidate may not be absorbed when taken with meals. Third, our pills are put into gelatin capsules, since the Ritalin placebo pills have a different tast (sweet) than the drug or active pills (bitter). Finally, for comparison of drug and placebo states, testing is done between 1 and 3 hours after medication.

It is important to note that each child is seen on 2 successive days for the evaluation of the acute response to stimulant medication. We have found that 1 day is insufficient for at least two reasons: (1) On the initial day, the child to be tested is often apprehensive and nervous, and his behavior and performance on our tests may not represent his usual condition, which is associated with his current problem; and (2) The first day is necessary to determine the level of difficulty for testing each particular child, which will avoid a ceiling or a floor effect. The initial testing is also necessary to provide practice on the test, which acts to stabilize performance on the next day.

In our research, each patient is assigned one of the following four orders of drug (D) or placebo (P) administration across the 2 days:

	Day 1		*Day 2*	
	A.M.	*P.M.*	*A.M.*	*P.M.*
Order 1	D	P	D	P
Order 2	D	P	P	D
Order 3	P	D	P	D
Order 4	P	D	D	P

We realize that a slight residual drug effect may occur in the afternoon when the drug is given in the morning.

The Patient Population

All subjects of the laboratory investigations are patients of the Learning Clinic of the Hospital for Sick Children. Children are referred to the Learning Clinic by parents, teachers, and pediatricians. Parent and teacher questionnaires are obtained for each child and are interpreted before the initial clinic visit.

The initial clinic visit is used to obtain a detailed history from the parent and to perform a general and neurologic examination of the child. The child returns later for a detailed psychological assessment in order to obtain information on his or her level of intelligence and achievement.

The pediatrician uses all the data gathered from the sources listed above to determine if the patient has symptoms that suggest hyperactivity. Enough has been written about the symptoms of the hyperactive child. The earlier descriptions[9,11] are excellent and, given the availability of more recent descriptions,[2,3,6,24] no detailed description will be provided here. About 40% of the patients referred to the learning clinic are tentatively diagnosed as hyperactive, and only those receive our laboratory tests.

Conners[13,14] has determined norms for his parent and teacher questionnaires which indicate that a score of over 15 on each questionnaire (or over 30 on the two combined) represents an abnormally high score, in that it amounts to two standard deviations above the mean for a normal control group. We[25] have recently obtained background information on our clinical population by using the Conners questionnaires. In a sample of 48 children referred with symptoms of hyperactivity, one-third had scores of over 15 on both parent and teacher rating scales, one-third had scores of over 15 on only the parent rating scale, and one-third had scores of over 15 on only the teacher rating scale.

Published Research Using the 2-Day Paradigm

At the present time, four studies have been published or accepted for publication. Swanson and Kinsbourne[20] describe state-dependent learning in hyperactive children treated with stimulants; Swanson, Kinsbourne, Roberts, and Zucker[26] describe the length of action of both favorable and adverse responders to methylphenidate; Dalby, Kinsbourne, Swanson, and Sobol[27] present data on the concentration span of hyperactive children in drug and placebo conditions; and Humphries, Kinsbourne, and Swanson[28] describe how stimulant medication affects the interaction of hyperactive children and their mothers. The first three studies used the paired-associate learning test to document the acute drug effect. The last used a mother–child interaction task for the same purpose.

The paired-associate learning task was the primary behavioral task of our early research on this topic, and it has remained the primary task for our clinical applications and our later research. Because of its importance in our research program, it will be described in detail below.

The paired-associate learning task was selected because (1) performance on it has been found to have a positive and highly significant correlation with performance in the classroom,[29] (2) it can be used to test repeatedly with little practice effect (or transfer) emerging over time when arranged appropriately,[30] and (3) it has been used successfully to measure the effect of an acute administration of stimulant medication.[31] In our paired-associate task, pictures of animals in naturalistic settings are used as stimuli, and the four directions (north, south, east, and west) are used as responses. Since there are more stimuli than responses, the task involves assigning stimuli (animals) to classes (directions).

A particular learning session consists of presenting a list of stimulus items (animal pictures), one at a time in a random sequence, for the patient to see and study. During the initial presentation of a list (which could be from 4 to 10 items long, depending on the patient's capacity as determined on the first day), the patient is told verbally to associate each animal with one of four hypothetical "zoos"—the North Zoo, the South Zoo, the East Zoo, or the West Zoo.

Starting on the second time through the list, the patient is asked to say in which zoo each animal lives. If the patient's first response is incorrect, a second response is allowed. If the second response is also incorrect, the correct response is provided verbally to reinstruct the patient as to which association was appropriate. The list is presented 10 times, each time in a random order, or until a criterion of two perfect recitations of the list is met. To accomplish this, the subject must concentrate on the task for about 15 minutes while sitting in the same place (a chair) and listening to an adult experimenter/teacher provide new information regarding the association to be made between old and familiar items. The cognitive skills necessary for much of the learning in the traditional classroom, including the ability to persevere at a task imposed by an adult, are necessary to perform this task.

How can one choose a task such that a practice effect will not occur from list to list? From the study of human learning in the psychology laboratory, "transfer" characteristic of different list structures have been determined. In the jargon of experimental psychology, the list sequence utilized in this experiment is labeled "A-B–C-B", to denote that the stimulus items change across lists but the response items do not. As reviewed by Kausler,[30] the stimulus aspects of the list structure (common zoo animals, which change from list to list) produce slight negative transfer, but the unchanging response set produces slight positive transfer. The two transfer effects, which are opposite in direction, are thought to be equal in magnitude, so virtually no overall transfer from list to list is to be expected. Other list structures are expected to result in either overall positive or overall negative transfer, as noted by Kausler[30] (Table 5.3) and thus would contaminate the time-response characteristics of the patient's performance following drug administration. The particular list structure utilized in this experiment is specially designed so that the assumption of equal task difficulty across time can reasonably be expected to hold.

State-Dependent Learning

An important question about any drug treatment concerns its long-term effect. If a drug is used to induce a short-term therapeutic effect on a patient, will that beneficial effect last when the drug treatment is stopped? Miller[32] voiced the concern that drug benefits may not be permanent because of state-dependent effects. State dependency has been demonstrated in numerous experiments on animals, most elegantly in a series of experiments by Overton[33] in the context of learning. If a task is learned when a drug treatment has been given, and then a test for retention is given later when a second drug treatment has been given, one can measure how much was remembered. However, if the drug treatment is withheld during the first (learning) test, then performance on the retention test is observed to suffer relative to the other combination of learning and retention states when the drug is given both times. A similar condition exists when the retention test occurs in a non drug (placebo) state: if retention is tested in the same state as learning (a placebo-placebo combination), then performance is better than if different states exist in the learning and retention tests (a drug–placebo combination).

This work on animals has important implications for drug therapy in humans. If a long-term effect is desired, then a short-term drug treatment may be useless if its effects are limited to a temporary drug-induced state. Our first experiment demonstrated that state-dependent learning can indeed be demonstrated in the laboratory in the context of the treatment of hyperactive children with the stimulant drug methylphenidate. The organization of the learning test is described in Figure 1. As shown there, initial learning in the paired-associate learning task takes place in two conditions during the first day; at one time the patient is in a drug state, and at the other time the patient is in a placebo state. On the second day, half of the material learned in the placebo state is combined with half of the material learned in the drug state, to provide one list for testing retention; the remaining material is also combined for a second retention test.

On the second day, drug and placebo states are again established, and a retention test is given in each state. As shown in Figure 1, half of the material presented for retention on each test on the

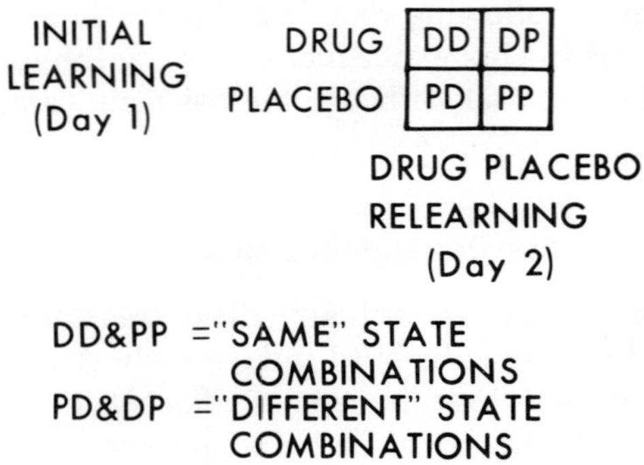

Figure 1. Design for the state-dependent learning experiment.

second day had been initially learned in the same state as the test state, and half of the material had been learned in the opposite state. The four combinations of learning and retention state (drug–drug, placebo–drug, placebo–placebo, drug–placebo) which are obtained from this design can be used to evaluate state-dependent learning.

The results of our laboratory test are presented in Figure 2, which shows that the same-state combinations result in much better performance than the different-state combinations of learning and retention states. Note that, even though an overall drug-induced

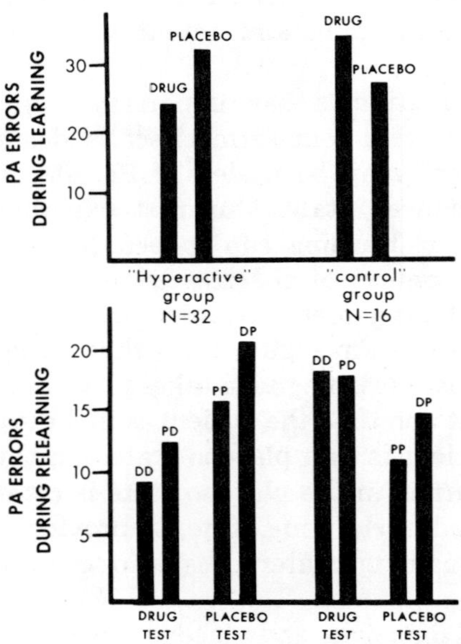

Figure 2. Results of the state-dependent learning experiment. Adapted from Swanson and Kinsbourne.[20]

improvement is apparent, it is counteracted if the initial learning took place in the placebo state. And more important, note that if learning takes place in the drug state and then testing is given in the placebo state, performance is worse than if the drug treatment is never given.

Thus it is apparent that, at least in our laboratory tests, the beneficial effects of the drug on cognitive performance occur in only one of the four learning retention combinations: the drug–drug combination. If the drug treatment is given inconsistently, then either no overall effect is observed in the placebo–drug combination, or a drug-induced impairment is observed in the drug–placebo combination.

Time–Response Characteristics of a Single Dose

Based on the behavior of hyperactive children taking methylphenidate, parents and teachers have consistently reported that the drug has an effective length of action of about 4 hours. Our second experiment was designed to determine the effective length of action on cognitive behavior in the laboratory. In this experiment, we used the same type of paired-associate learning test that we developed for the state-dependent learning task, but we gave only the learning phase of the test, repeatedly over an 8-hour period on the second of the 2 days of testing.

On the first day, the list length appropriate for each subject's capacity was determined by starting with a list of four items, and then increasing the list by two items if a criterion of two errorless recitations of the list was achieved within 12 trials. This procedure was continued until the list was increased to the point that the criterion could not be met, or until the maximum list length of ten items was reached. The capacity list length was defined for each subject as the longest list for which the criterion was attained.

The list length determined on Day 1 was adhered to when eight different lists of the same length were presented on the second day. The eight tests were distributed across the 8 hours of testing between 8:30 A.M. and 4:30 P.M., so as to sample performance throughout the periods of expected drug action. All testing was conducted under double-blind conditions. The testing times were as follows:

8:30 A.M.	before administration I
9:30	½ hour after administration I
11:00	2 hours after administration I
12:00	3 hours after administration I
12:45 P.M.	½ hour after administration II
2:15	2 hours after administration II

3:15 3 hours after administration II
4:15 3 hours after administration II

Results

The results of our testing are presented in Table 1 and Figures 3 and 4. The primary purpose of this research was to monitor the time course of the effect of methylphenidate, but before that could be accomplished, the pattern (favorable or adverse) of response had to be specified for each individual. The procedures and the criteria for this initial classification of adverse and favorable responders are presented elsewhere.[26] Contingent upon this separation, the time characteristics of the two patterns of response were delineated, characterizing these two patterns of response to medication.

As shown in Figure 3, two types of responses were clearly defined. The favorable response resulted in a decrease in errors on the learning task by 2 hours after medication, and the adverse response resulted in an increase in errors on the learning task by 2 hours after the drug treatment. Approximately two-thirds of the patients had a favorable response to the drug on the basis of this laboratory test, which is the same as the percentage reported in the literature on the basis of clinical judgment.

What are the initial differences in the groups of favorable and adverse responders? First, as shown in Table 1, the favorable re-

TABLE 1
Group Means for Performance on the Paired-associate Learning Task. (Scores Reflect Percentage Change in Errors from Baseline.)

	Favorable Responders		*Adverse Responders*	
	Drug–Placebo (n = 10)	*Placebo–Drug (n = 13)*	*Drug–Placebo (n = 7)*	*Placebo–Drug (n = 9)*
Group averages on Initial (baseline) Test	39.4 ± 4.3	27.3 ± 2.2	22.6 ± 2.8	24.8 ± 6.0
8:45 A.M.	0 (baseline)	0 (baseline)	0 (baseline)	0 (baseline)
9:30 A.M.	−36.7[a]	0.0	17.7	9.8
11:00 A.M.	−49.6[a]	+14.3	52.2[a]	18.3
12:00 Noon	−39.1[a]	+67.1[a]	67.8[a]	26.3
12:45 P.M.	−43.4[a]	+ 0.7	21.3	45.3[a]
2:15 P.M.	−42.1[a]	−26.7[b]	5.3	46.7[a]
3:15 P.M.	−36.5[a]	−24.7	44.1[a]	28.6[b]
4:15 P.M.	−25.6	6.7	26.7[b]	67.3[a]

[a] $p < 0.01$; confidence interval = 0 ± 35.1.
[b] $p < 0.05$; confidence interval = 0 ± 26.6.

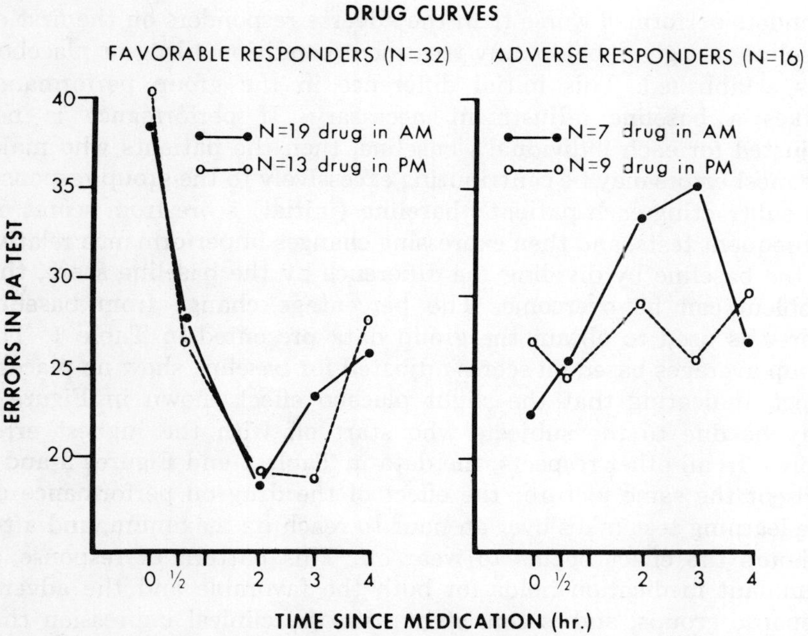

Figure 3. Time–response curves showing the effect of a single dose of methylphenidate. Adapted from Swanson et al.[26]

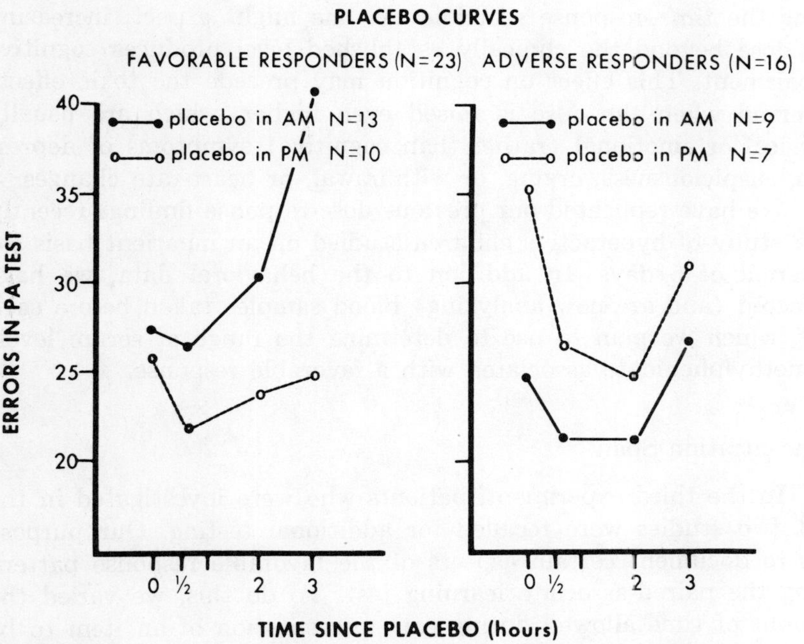

Figure 4. Placebo curves from the time–response study. Adapted from Swanson et al.[26]

sponders performed worse than the adverse responders on the first or baseline test given before any treatment condition (drug or placebo) was established. This initial difference in the group performance makes a baseline adjustment necessary. If performance is not adjusted for each individual's baseline, then the patients who make the most errors may be contributing excessively to the group response. By subtracting each patient's baseline (initial) score from scores on subsequent tests, and then expressing changes in performance relative to the baseline by dividing the difference by the baseline score, this problem can be overcome. The percentage change from baseline scores as used to obtain the group data presented in Table 1. The group averages based on scores adjusted for baseline show no placebo effect, indicating that the slight placebo effect shown in Figure 4 may be due to the subjects who start off with the highest error scores. In all other respects, the data in Table 1 and Figures 3 and 4 present the same picture: the effect of the drug on performance on the learning test takes over an hour to reach its maximum, and after 2 hours the effect begins to wear off. This pattern of response to stimulant medication holds for both the favorable and the adverse response groups, and is consistent with the clinical impression that methylphenidate has an effective length of action of about 4 hours.

In our previous work, we reported a dose–response curve for five patients who were retested on an optimal and excessive dose using the time–response schedule. As one might expect, increasing the dose beyond the clinically established level produces cognitive impairment. This effect on cognition may precede the toxic effects observed when the dose is raised even higher, which are usually physical or emotional (rather than cognitive) symptoms of depression, suspiciousness, crying, or withdrawal, or heart-rate changes.

We have replicated our previous dose-response findings recently in a study of hyperactive children studied on an inpatient basis for a period of 5 days. In addition to the behavioral data, we have collected (and are now analyzing) blood samples taken before each test, which we plan to use to determine the range of serum levels of methylphenidate associated with a favorable response.

Concentration Span

In the third experiment, patients who were investigated in the first two studies were recalled for additional testing. Our purpose was to document certain aspects of the favorable response pattern using the paired-associate learning test. To do this, we varied the amount of time allowed during each presentation of an item to be learned in order to determine if hyperactive children failed to take advantage of long time intervals as effectively as they took advantage of short time intervals.

As shown in Figure 5, we set up conditions which allowed 4, 8, or 12 seconds per item for learning. According to the "total-time hypothesis," developed from performance of normal college students, the prediction was made that a few long intervals (e.g., four 12-second presentations) would result in the same amount of learning as many short intervals (e.g., twelve 4-second presentations). However, hyperactive patients did not take advantage of the long intervals effectively, and thus in the placebo state performed relatively poorly in the condition in which each trial was relatively lengthy. This pattern of performance is abnormal, for the total-time hypothesis has been shown to hold for both normal adults and normal children in a variety of settings. As Figure 5 also indicates, the effect of the drug treatment was to improve the favorable responder's utilization of the long intervals and to impair the performance of the adverse responders (who had been identified on the basis of previous laboratory tests).

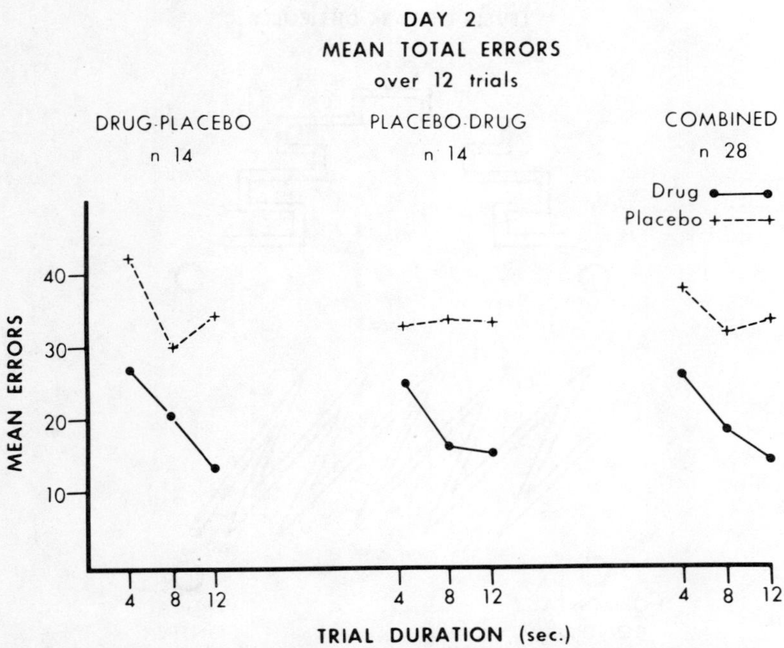

Figure 5. The total-time relationship in the performance of hyperactive children on a learning test. From Dalby et al.[27]

Since the items we presented for learning were available for only a short time (under 12 seconds in all cases), we have demonstrated that the hyperactive child finds it hard to concentrate for more than brief periods. Our data show that the concentration span of the children in the placebo state was under 8 seconds, since at that presentation rate a deficit (failure to take full advantage of the learning time offered) was already present. Our data also show that the effect of the drug was to increase the concentration span of our patients to over 12 seconds.

Mother–Child Interactions

The fourth experiment in our research program measured the drug effect in another way. To determine how mothers and their hyperactive children could cooperate, we set up a task using a toy called the Etch-a-Sketch (Fig. 6). This toy has two dials which control a marker which can be used to draw a path on a rectangular screen. We put a target on the face of the Etch-a-Sketch, and asked

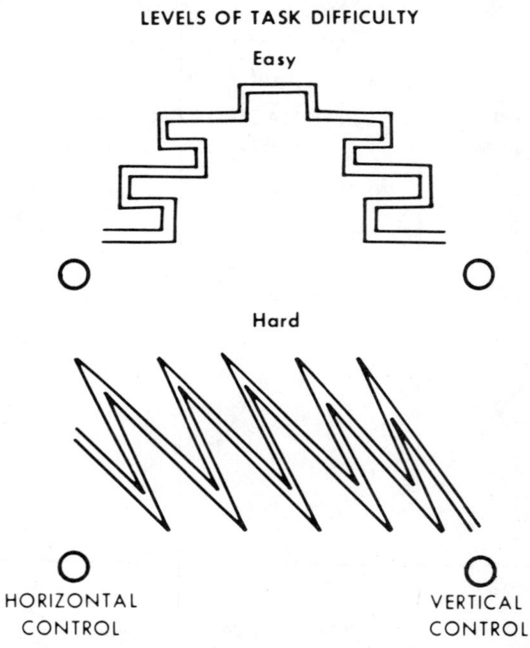

Figure 6. Types of mazes used on the Etch-a-Sketch to obtain mother–child interaction in the laboratory. From Humphries et al.[28]

the mother and child to draw a line through the target path, with the child controlling one dial and the mother the other dial.

As the two performed this task, their interactions in terms of verbal communication, praise, and criticism, were noted. As shown in Table 2, performance on the task (in terms of errors made and time taken to complete the path) improved in the drug condition relative to the placebo condition. In addition to these measures of performance, the following pattern of changes in verbal interaction was noted:

When the hyperactive children were in a medicated as opposed to a placebo state, they and their mothers praised each other more and criticized each other less; the mothers gave fewer directions to their children about how to complete the task, and the children gave more directions to their mothers. Since some mothers and their children performed at a faster pace in the drug condition than the placebo condition, while others performed more slowly when the children were on medication, there was no significant difference in the time taken to complete the task for the drug and placebo states.

The finding that some mothers and their children increased the pace of their performance in the drug condition, while others reverted to a slower pace, raises the possibility that certain of the hyperactive children in this study may have differed in the degree to which they are distractible versus impulsive. Results from the Etch-a-Sketch task, and several other tasks in our laboratory that

TABLE 2
Means and Standard Errors of Interaction Variables on Maze I and Maze II in Placebo and Drug Conditions

	Placebo				*Drug*			
	Maze I		*Maze II*		*Maze I*		*Maze II*	
Variable	M	SE	M	SE	M	SE	M	SE
Time	147.27	7.04	331.50	26.72	147.62	5.36	352.58	35.55
Errors	2.69	0.77	20.73	3.10	1.19	0.30	9.42	2.52
Mothers' directions	6.77	1.48	20.19	2.68	2.96	0.69	8.08	1.65
Children's directions	1.58	0.31	5.81	1.26	3.77	0.62	11.19	2.88
Mothers' praise	0.19	0.10	0.23	0.13	0.54	0.24	0.96	0.25
Children's praise	0.00	0.00	0.08	0.08	0.38	0.13	0.65	0.33
Mothers' criticism	0.69	0.21	2.31	0.60	0.00	0.00	0.12	0.08
Children's criticism	0.58	0.21	2.92	0.49	0.04	0.04	0.31	0.13

hyperactive children perform alone, have revealed that some children who are easily distracted, slow to respond, and frequently inaccurate in their response when in an unmedicated state, respond faster but more accurately on the drug. Other hyperactive children respond impulsively, and therefore often erroneously when off drug, respond more slowly and also more correctly when medicated.

This differential effect that stimulant medication has on the style of responding of hyperactive children whose behavior varies along an impulsivity–distractibility dimension, suggests that a similar difference in cognitive styles could have existed for the hyperactive children in the present study, and thereby accounted for the two contrasting patterns of task completion times observed in the drug condition.

This study demonstrates how a mother's felt need for control over her hyperactive child can be significantly reduced by a single, acute administration of stimulant medication (methylphenidate) to the child. Furthermore, this "normalizing" of the interaction between mothers and their hyperactive children was obtained not only for relevant aspects of social interaction, but also on a performance measure that investigated the effectiveness of the mothers and their children in working as a team to achieve a common goal.

This study of mother–child interaction marks a change in our research program. As the first three studies indicate, our initial emphasis has been on the learning ability of hyperactive children. We have now extended that narrow focus to include different aspects of behavior. Several other studies have been conducted to provide information on the effect of stimulant drugs on various aspects of behavior.

Additional Studies

In the course of our research, we have continued to use the paired-associate learning task to separate favorable and adverse responders to stimulant treatment. We have also observed the performance of these two groups of patients on several other measures of performance in order to further characterize the acute response to stimulants.

We[34] have used a laboratory computer (a DECLAB 11/40 system) to present a moving target (an octagon) on a display screen which the patient watches. The patient's task is to keep a dot centered inside the target by using a control stick which moves the dot. We gave each patient a target size adjusted for his level of competence, and measured the accuracy of performance 100 times/

second so we could observe even momentary lapses in performance. A patient performs the tracking task for 40 seconds, rests for 10 seconds, and then performs the task again until 10 trials are completed.

Performance on that task declines across the 10 trials. This type of decline is not unusual, and in the literature is called a *vigilance decrement*. It occurs in normal adults performing this task, as well as in both the favorable and adverse responders who compose our population of patients. We have observed the effect of the drug treatment on the two groups of patients defined by their opposite response to drug (favorable or adverse) on the learning test.

In the first day of testing in our 2-day paradigm, only the group of favorable responders show an improvement in performance in the drug relative to the placebo condition. On the second day, however, both groups show better performance in the drug condition. It is possible on a task such as this, which requires maintenance of attention over time, that a stimulant drug would improve the performance of anyone. If this is the case, then the diagnostic utility of this task may be limited, since an improvement on medication would occur for normal (i.e., nonhyperactive) children as well as hyperactive children.

A similar result has been obtained when the Continuous Performance Task is used in the context of the 2-day drug trial.[35] When patients are required to monitor a slide presentation for the occurrence of a particular number, their performance in terms of errors and reaction time to the critical number is better in the drug than in the placebo condition. This pattern has been found to hold for patients who are labeled as adverse responders, on the basis of tests on the paired-associate learning task, as well as for the favorable responders.

The computer-controlled tracking task and the Continuous Performance Task both are designed to induce boredom due to the repetitive and uninteresting nature of the tasks. In those tasks, both hyperactive children and normal adults show a decline in performance over time (the vigilance decrement) and a drug-induced improvement when stimulants are given. To determine what happens when a more complex and interesting task is presented, we used the Matching Familiar Figures Test. We separated children not only according to their response to the drug based on paired-associate learning performance, but also according to whether their clinical history was chiefly one of impulsivity or distractibility.

In the Matching Familiar Figures Test (MFF), a patient must inspect a standard figure and then pick it out from an array of six to eight similar figures. The latency before the first response is considered a measure of cognitive style on the dimension of impulsivity/reflectivity, and the number of errors made before choosing the correct figure is taken as an accuracy measure.

Mock, Swanson, and Kinsbourne[36] have found that the effect of the drug on latency of response depends on the type of patient: the drug induces the impulsive patients to slow down and the distractible patients to speed up. The overall effect of the drug on MFF latency measures taken from both types of hyperactive children is essentially zero. The population must be divided into two subgroups (distractible and impulsive) before the drug effect can be predicted. In terms of the error score, the drug produces the same effect on performance on the MFF task as it does on the paired-associate learning (PAL) task. The patients who respond favorably on the PAL task decrease errors on the MFF task in the drug versus the placebo condition, and the patient who responds adversely on the PAL task increase errors on the MFF task in the drug condition.

Thus, in the evaluated groups, one measure of performance on the MFF task is sensitive to drug effects (the error score), but the other is not (the latency score).

Freeman[37] has used the Lykken Mazé to document the effect of stimulants on avoidance learning. This task requires a child to choose among four alternative "paths" at each of 20 choice points to find the way through a complex maze. At each point, one choice is correct and three are wrong. One of the three incorrect choices is associated with punishment—a noxious auditory stimulus. We have found that hyperactive children do as well as controls on overall performance on this task, but that they make a large percentage of errors that are "punished" than do the controls. This indicates that the normal strategy of avoiding punishment is not adopted by hyperactive children. By testing the hyperactive children in drug and placebo conditions, Freeman[37] has reported that the percentage of punished errors made on the task is lower in the drug than in the Placebo condition. Thus, the abnormal performance in the placebo condition seems to have been normalized in the drug condition.

Knowledge of Drug and Placebo States

We have tested several hundred children using our 2-day, double-blind procedure. We have been aware that, despite large differences in performance on our tests, the children we test do not seem to know when they receive the "real pill" (medication) and when they receive the "fake pill" (placebo). Over a period of time we asked 121 successive patients tested in the laboratory to tell us, after the 2 days of drug–placebo administration described earlier, which pill on each day was medication and which was placebo. The data we collected were consistent with our informal observations: 78 of the 121 patients were favorable responders on our tests, but only 52% of their answers concerning the drug state were correct. The remaining 43 were adverse responders on our tests, but only 58% of their answers were correct when we inquired about the drug and placebo conditions. Thus, neither the favorable nor the adverse responders to medication could differentiate between the drug and placebo states.

This information is important because it confirms what is generally thought about stimulant therapy: at the doses used to treat hyperactive children, there is no strong feeling of euphoria or well-being experienced by the patients that identifies the drug treatment as a pleasurable experience to be repeated. The pleasurable subjective effect apparently felt by those drug abusers who take large doses of stimulant drugs is not experienced by the hyperactive children, who cannot even tell when they receive the drug in low doses. The lack of a subjective effect may be why there is no problem of addiction to stimulant drugs in the population of hyperactive children who have been given the drug for the medical treatment of hyperactivity.

Follow Up Studies

At this stage in our research program, we have developed a number of tasks that could potentially be used for distinguishing those children referred for hyperactivity who would do well on stimulant therapy from those who would do poorly. After a single administration of methylphenidate, some of our patients improved their test performance; others did worse. However, merely by increasing the dose, a favorable response can be transformed into an adverse response in the same child. How do these acute laboratory responses relate to long-term outcome?

The task that we have explored most thoroughly to date is the paired-associate learning test. We have an abundance of clinical information suggesting that when a favorable response to stimulants occurs on this task, the child is very likely to do well in the longer term. However, the diagnostic utility of other tasks which we have tried (e.g., the tracking task or the continuous performance task) has not been established.

In a recent follow-up study[38] 42 patients who had been taking stimulant medication for over 6 months were recalled for the usual reevaluation by a pediatrician to assess response to medication. At the same time, we gave our learning test to evaluate response to a single dose of medication compared to a placebo condition. The pediatrician made a clinical judgment in each case as to whether the patient taking stimulants should stay on medication or discontinue it. A similar judgment was made on the basis of performance in the drug and placebo conditions.

Of the 42 patients, 36 were males. In these 36 boys, the laboratory tests and the clinical judgments were consistent on 28 (78 percent). However, the clinical judgments and laboratory tests were in agreement for only 2 of the 6 girls, (33 percent).

This information suggests that our laboratory learning test provides a way of confirming a diagnosis of hyperactivity based on a diagnostic drug trial, but whether the additional information provided by the laboratory tests may be of value for females, requires further study with a greater number of patients.

The proposition that children who respond adversely to stimulants in the laboratory would also do so in the longer term is more difficult to validate clinically. We have not been inclined to risk prescribing medication which caused adverse acute effects in the laboratory, but others have suggested that an initial adverse effect does not always indicate a similar long-term effect. In the future, we hope to provide some systematic evidence on this matter, but at the present time, we do not have the data to make a decision about what the outcome of adverse responders would be on long-term stimulant medication. However, we do know that for male favorable responders, the acute diagnostic drug trial and the long-term diagnostic drug trial (evaluated by a trained pediatrician) yield consistent results.

The Theoretical Utility of Laboratory Testing

The primary purpose of the research program described in this paper is to provide information on the performance of hyperactive children in classical paradigms from experimental psychology. The information we have obtained, for example, on state-dependent learning and the total-time hypothesis, is relevant to the general theory of learning as well as valuable in the study of hyperactivity. We have discussed the theoretical significance of our work in the separate articles which are available in the literature.

The secondary purpose of our research program is to improve

the clinical treatment of hyperactive children. We hope that our research will have practical value. The experience to date on how our laboratory tests have been used in a clinical setting will be discussed below.

The Clinical Utility of Laboratory Testing

The laboratory tests we have described in this chapter are not easy to give. The testing procedure is long (at least four tests spread across 2 days), and each test must be individually administered and takes about 20–40 minutes, depending on the patient's ability and cooperation. What is the clinical benefit of this difficult and time-consuming procedure?

First, we should make clear that our laboratory testing is not designed to replace the traditional examination and clinical treatment of hyperactive children. Instead, our testing provides additional information for the pediatrician, who, based on the usual information derived from medical examination, psychological testing, and consultation with parents and teachers, may still be uncertain about whether to initiate or continue stimulant drug therapy in a particular child. A review of the use of our laboratory methods in the Learning Clinic of the Hospital for Sick Children will demonstrate how they are applied in a clinical setting. Children referred with symptoms of hyperactivity are initially seen by a pediatrician in the Clinic. After a physical and neurologic examination, a detailed history is taken from the parent. Information on school performance is obtained before the Clinic visit. Based on all the available information, a list of critical symptoms which may suggest hyperactivity is made by the pediatrician. Over the past 2 years, symptoms of hyperactivity have been observed in about 40 percent of the patients referred to our clinic.

If symptoms of hyperactivity are documented in this initial screening, a diagnostic drug trial is indicated. However, before a long-term trial in the home and school setting is tried, an acute laboratory is trial is given. The purpose of this initial trial in the laboratory is to provide confirming (or nonconfirming) information to the pediatrician concerning his provisional diagnosis of hyperactivity. Over the past 2 years, approximately 65% of the clinic patients who had symptoms of hyperactivity and were tested with our laboratory tasks actually had a favorable response to the short drug trial. All these children (the favorable responders) and a few of the others were then given a traditional long-term diagnostic drug trial. Follow-up information was obtained by telephone over the next 4–6 weeks, and a normal follow-up with a Clinic visit was performed between 6 and 12 months later. At the time of the follow-up in the Clinic, most of the patients were retested in the laboratory.

The laboratory testing described in this chapter is an adjunct to the standard program used by many clinicians, which emphasizes the treatment of hyperactive children with stimulant drugs. The information derived from our laboratory testing is used by the pediatrican to confirm a diagnosis of hyperactivity. This, of course, is in accord with the logical procedure described by Laufer and Denhoff[11] years ago, and is new only with regard to how the information is obtained.

Our laboratory procedure provides valuable additional information to the pediatrician. First, our testing shows the direct effect of drug treatment on the patient, which is more accurate than a report from an adult on that effect. In some cases, reports from parents or teachers may describe the favorable effects of the drug treatment on those who have to deal with the patient rather than the effects of treatment on the patient himself. Our laboratory tests allow the pediatrician to confirm or deny the subjective evaluation of parents and teachers.

Second, we test cognitive ability, not conduct. It is clear that stimulant medication affects both cognition and conduct,[39] but the measurement of the cognitive effect is more difficult than that of the effect on conduct, which may be obtained from parent and teacher questionnaires.

Finally, our tests can be given over a short period in a controlled setting, so other factors that may confuse the outcome of a long-term drug trial can be excluded or held constant in the laboratory.

Summary

The methods used for initiating and maintaining stimulant therapy for hyperactive children are almost as numerous as the physicians who use this form of symptomatic treatment. This is a clear indication that proper guidelines are not available. The level of initial dosage, the pattern of subsequent dosage if the initial attempt is judged ineffective, and the nature of feedback as to outcome (evidence from parent interview, telephone conversation, questionnaire) vary widely. The consequences are that one learns little from the information that stimulants have been tried (elsewhere) and worked, or that they were tried and did not work. The laboratory procedures we have developed exemplify a systematic approach to the implementation of stimulant therapy. While our methods have not yet been readied for general use, they were developed with this goal in mind. Once we have sufficiently stablished the reliability and validity of these techniques, we plan to modify them to make them available for use elsewhere.

References

1. Bradley, C.: The behavior of children receiving benzedrine. *Am J. Psychiatry* **94:** 577, 1937.
2. Wender, P.: *Minimal Brain Dysfunction in Children.* Wiley, New York, 1971.
3. Cantwell, D.P.: *The Hyperactive Child: Diagnosis, Management, Current Research.* Spectrum Publications, Holliswood, New York, 1975.
4. Safer, D.S., and Allen, R.P.: *Hyperactive Children: Diagnosis and Management.* University Park Press, Baltimore, 1976.
5. Barkley, R.A.: A review of stimulant drug research with hyperactive children. *J. Child Psychol Psychiatry* **18:** 137, 1977.
6. Kinsbourne, M.: The mechanism of hyperactivity. In *Topics in Child Neurology,* M. Blau, I. Rapin, and M. Kinsbourne, Eds. Spectrum Press, New York, 1977.
7. Grinspoon, L., and Hedbloom, B.: *The Speed Culture.* Harvard University Press, Cambridge, 1975.
8. Schmitt, B.D.: The minimal brain dysfunction myth. *Am J Dis Child* **129:** 1313, 1975.
9. Bradley, C.: Benzedrine and Dexedrine in the treatment of children's behavior disorders. *Pediatrics* **5:** 24, 1950.
10. Eisenberg, L.: The clinical use of stimulant drugs in children. *Pediatrics* **49:** 709, 1972.
11. Laufer, M., and Denhoff, E. Hyperactive behavior symptoms in children. *J Pediatr* **50:** 463, 1957.
12. Solomons, G.: Guidelines on the use and medical effects of psychostimulant drugs in therapy. *J Learn Disord* **5:** 6, 1971.
13. Conners, C.K.: A teacher rating scale for use in drug studies with children. *Am J Psychiatry* **126:** 884, 1969.
14. Conners, C.K.: Rating scales for use in drug studies with children. *Psychopharmacol Bull* (Special Issue) **24:** 1973.
15. Schain, R.J., and Reynard, C.L.: Observations and effects of a central stimulant drug (methylphenidate) on children with hyperactive behavior. *Pediatrics* **55:** 709, 1975.
16. Conners, C.K.: Physiological effects of stimulant drugs in children with minimal brain dysfunction. *Pediatrics* **49:** 702, 1972.
17. Report of the Conference on the Use of Stimulant Drugs in the Treatment of Behaviorally Disturbed Young School Children. Office of Child Development and Office of the Assistant Secretary for Health and Scientific Affairs, Dept. of Health and Welfare, January 11–12, 1971.
18. Grinspoon, L., and Singer, B.: Amphetamines as the treatment for hyperactive children. *Harvard Ed Rev* **43:** 515, 1973.
19. Kinsbourne, M.: Personality of hyperactive children and stimulant therapy. Presented at the American Psychological Association Meeting, Montreal, 1973.
20. Swanson, J.M., and Kinsbourne, M.: Stimulant-related state-dependent learning in hyperactive children. *Science* **192:** 1754, 1976.
21. Kinsbourne, M., Roberts, W., and Swanson, J.: Stimulant-related state-dependent learning in hyperactive children: The effect of first trial on medication. Presented at the Society for Pediatric Research Meeting, St. Louis, 1976.

22. Fish, B.: The one-child, one-drug myth. *Arch Gen Psychiatry* **25:** 193, 1971.
23. Yoss, R.E., and Daly, D.D.: On the treatment of narcolepsy. *Med Clin North Am* **52:** 781, 1968.
24. Douglas, V.I.: Stop, look and listen: The problem of sustained attention and impulse control in hyperactive and normal children. *Can J Behav Sci* **4:** 259, 1972.
25. Swanson, J.M., Fisher, J., and Kinsbourne, M.: On the use of questionnaires, achievement tests, and laboratory tests to document the effect of stimulant drugs on hyperactive children. (In preparation.)
26. Swanson, J.M., Kinsbourne, M., Roberts, W., and Zucker, K.: A time-response analysis of the effect of stimulant medication on the learning ability of children referred for hyperactivity. *Pediatrics* **61**:21, 1978.
27. Dalby, T., Kinsbourne, M., Swanson, J.M., and Sobol, M.: Hyperactive children's underuse of learning time. *Child Dev* (in press).
28. Humphries, T., Kinsbourne, M., and Swanson, J.M.: Stimulant effects on co-operation and social interaction between hyperactive children and their mothers. *J Child Psychol Psychiatry* **19**:13, 1978.
29. Stevenson, H.W.: *Children's Learning*. Appleton-Century-Crofts, New York, 1972.
30. Kausler, D.H.: *Psychology of Verbal Learning and Memory*. Academic Press, New York, 1974.
31. Conners, C.K., Eisenberg, L., and Sharpe, L.: Effects of methylphenidate (Ritalin) on paired-associate learning and Porteus maze performance in emotionally disturbed children. *J Consult Psychol* **28:** 14, 1964.
32. Miller, N.E.: Some animal experiments pertinent to the problem of combining psychotherapy with drug therapy. *Compr Psychiatry* **7:** 1, 1966.
33. Overton, D.A.: Methods for the study of state-dependent learning. *Fed Proc* **33:** 1800, 1974.
34. Kapelus, G., Swanson, J.M., and Kinsbourne, M.: Effects of stimulant drugs on the performance of hyperactive children on a computer controlled tracking task. (In preparation.)
35. Barlow, A.: A neuropsychological study of a symptom of minimal brain dysfunction: Distractibility under levels of high and low stimulation. Ph.D. Thesis, University of Toronto, 1977.
36. Mock, K., Swanson, J.M., and Kinsbourne, M.: Performance of impulsive and distractible hyperactive children on the MFF task. (In preparation.)
37. Freeman, R.: A study of avoidance learning and risk taking in hyperactive children. Ph.D. Thesis, University of Waterloo, 1977.
38. Swanson, J.M., Serfontain, G., and Kinsbourne, M.: Confirming the diagnosis of stimulant responsive hyperactivity with a laboratory drug trial. (In preparation.)
39. Sprague, R.L., and Sleator, E.K.: What is the proper dose of stimulant drugs in children? *Int J Men Health* **4:** 75, 1975.

8

Controlled Studies of Efficacy of Long-Term Treatment with Stimulants of Hyperactive Children

Gabrielle Weiss, M.D.

Results of Acute Drug Studies

Over the last 15 years a series of well-controlled studies have conclusively demonstrated that some stimulant drugs, such as dextroamphetamine and methylphenidate improve certain aspects of behavior and cognitive function in a certain percentage of disturbed and hyperactive children, thus confirming Bradley's finding of 1937 that in a group of disturbed children Benzedrine improved the school performance and behavior of many of the children and had a paradoxical quietening effect on hyperactive children.[1] We now have more information as to the kinds of behavior and cognitive tasks which are affected by stimulants. With respect to behavior, we know that aggression[2] is reduced and that purposeless activity becomes more goal-directed.[3–6] With respect to cognitive tasks, we know that children on medication improve in tests of sustained attention,[7,8] are less impulsive,[9/12] learn rote material better,[9] have improved short-term memory,[10] do better on fine motor tasks,[11] and can better discriminate foreground from background.[12] It is not

Department of Psychiatry, McGill University and Montreal Childrens Hospital, Montreal, Quebec, Canada.

generally believed that stimulants improve perception, motor ability, or learning directly, but rather that these functions improve as a result of improved attention and an increase in reflectivity.

Extrapolation to Long-term Stimulant Drug Efficacy

Because no evidence appeared to the contrary and because clinical experience at first suggested that stimulants continue to be useful in improving the behavior of children when given over many years, it was taken for granted that stimulant drugs, whose efficacy had been demonstrated beyond a reasonable doubt in acute drug studies, would continue to be equally valuable if administered year after year. No reports appeared of tolerance developing to any of the behavioral or cognitive improvements, and the idea that tolerance might, in fact, take place to a varying degree (which might or might not be counteracted by dose increases) to my knowledge has not been seriously investigated.

However, several physicians, who were treating large numbers of hyperactive children in clinics with long-term stimulants, began to become more skeptical, particularly those who did not have adjunctive treatment programs such as behavior modification, family counseling, remedial education, etc. available for the children. Obviously too much had been expected from the use of stimulants and, for many, skepticism of long-term efficacy replaced the initial optimism that a "cure" had been found for the problems of hyperactive children. Many physicians had a large number of children in their practices who were on adequate doses of stimulants over several years, but who still had serious difficulties. Many of these children showed antisocial behavior, were behind in school, and were socially isolated and rejected. Clinically it was recognized by many that stimulants were helpful, but that hyperactive children, though somewhat improved, were far from trouble-free, and that other methods of rehabilitation in conjunction with or in place of stimulants were required.

Difficulties in the Design of Long-term Controlled Stimulant Drug Studies

For a controlled drug study there are two major techniques in common use. For the "within subject" design each child serves as his own control and receives an active drug and a placebo (or comparison drug) in random order. Serial testing for behavior and cognitive function is carried out. In the other common design children are randomly assigned to either an active drug group or a placebo (or comparison drug) group, and the groups are then matched on all parameters considered to be relevant to outcome, such as age, IQ, socioeconomic status, family pathology, severity of the condition, and so on. It is difficult to match children adequately on these sometimes subtle parameters. Yet it is in long-term studies that these very parameters are important. Both these designs have been used for long-term controlled studies, but there have been difficulties with both designs.

No investigator has found it possible to assign a child randomly to a stimulant or a no-treatment group for a period of several years. It is not ethical to withhold stimulants for years from children who might benefit from them, nor is it practical. Children would not stay for years (even if researchers wished them to) either on stimulants or without treatment. In practice, many children discontinue stimulant treatment for a large variety of reasons. The most obvious reason is that we know from the various acute drug studies that anywhere from 10 to 30 percent of children are not helped by stimulants. Second, children may, after taking the drug for a while, refuse to continue (other children tease them, they don't like the taste, they have side-effects, etc.). Perhaps most important of all, the benefits may decrease over time and, while the drug may still offer small advantages, parents may decide that the advantages are not worth the hazards, expense, nuisance, etc. Finally, children may stop needing stimulants, and hence slowly drop out of the drug group.

On the other hand, in designs where each child is his own control, only some questions about long-term stimulant drug efficacy are answered, for example, whether the child is better off with or without the active drug over the period of followup. The questions of long-term stimulant drug benefits have not been answered, for example, Are fewer grades failed? Do the stimulants help children not to become antisocial and rejected by their peers? We have to realize, unfortunately, that there is no way of designing and carrying out a perfect long-term drug efficacy study which would answer all the questions we want to ask.

One final note of caution concerning the assessment of outcome in long-term drug studies: in evaluating results one should take into account both the age at which stimulants were started and the age at which outcome was assessed. If stimulants are indeed to be effective in improving school performance, they should presumably be started before a child experiences accumulated school failures and the resultant loss of self-esteem. Hence, in an ideal long-term drug study, children should be started on stimulant by the time they are in the first grade. To include children who start on stimulants early and those children who are started on them only after years of school failure in one outcome group, and not to distinguish between them, may blur the results. In addition, the age of the child when outcome is assessed is also important. There is a natural history of the hyperactive syndrome, and studies have indicated that adolescence is a particularly difficult and turbulent time for hyperactive children.[13-15] Even if a stimulant drug is helpful in the preadolescent years, it will be particularly difficult to distinguish in adolescence between stimulant-treated hyperactives and hyperactives who were given no drugs. The florid symptoms of adolescence could well blur or mask subtle stimulant benefits which might only be detected either before or after adolescence.

A Critical Analysis of Three Controlled Long-Term Drug Studies

"Hyperactive Children: A Continuous Long-term Placebo Controlled Follow-up"[16]

The method of the study was as follows: the diagnosis of hyperkinesis was based on a combination of teachers' and parents' reports and the physician's evaluation. To be included in the study a child had to score 15 or above on the Conners Abbreviated Symptom Questionnaire. (Less than 2.5% of children in a classroom would fall in this group.) Children who did not respond well to stimulants (as assessed by a previous short-term double-blind crossover study of different mg/kg doses of methylphenidate) were excluded from the long-term follow-up study. Hence the 42 children who participated were all favorable responders to the drug.

During 1 month of the school year, with teacher, parent, and child "blind," a placebo was administered. At the end of each month throughout 2 years, the Conner Abbreviated Symptom Questionnaire (ASQ) was completed by each child's teacher, and the parents completed the Conners Parent Rating Scale. Some interesting findings emerged from this study.

First, teachers were more sensitive than parents in detecting when placebo was substituted for methylphenidate. In this study methylphenidate was given in the morning so that it is likely that effects had worn off by the time the child returned from school. Also, it is possible that the small doses used were insufficient to affect the "free play" situation of the home. It has been demonstrated in the same center (the Child Research and Development

Center, University of Illinois) that larger doses of methylphenidate are required to improve social behavior than tasks of cognitive function.

Another important observation was that only 40 percent of the children were rated by their teachers as being worse on placebo (17 of 42). Of the 17 patients who showed deterioration, 5 could not remain a whole month on placebo. It was noted that 26 percent of the whole group had stopped being any problem in the classroom within the first 1 to 2 years of observation, and they could be taken off stimulants. Finally, it was noted that 7 of the 17 children who became worse during the month on placebo required an increase in dosage for maintenance. That is, 41 percent of those who still needed stimulants required an increased dosage. It is not possible to know to what extent tolerance played a part in this. The study thus fails to answer the question of whether stimulants affect outcome measures in stimulant-treated versus non-stimulant-treated children.

"The Effect of Long-term Treatment of Hyperactive Children with Methylphenidate"[17]

At the Montreal Children's Hospital we conducted a study different in design to the one just discussed. We wanted to determine if the prognosis in adolescence was better for those children who had received methylphenidate for 3 to 5 years during elementary school compared with those treated with chlorpromazine for at least 18 months to 5 years and with those who had received no medication.

There were 24 children in the methylphenidate group, 22 in the chlorpromazine group, and 20 in the no-drug group. Initial IQ's were 105, 102, and 97 respectively (NS); initial ages were 7.9, 8.1, and 8.2 years (NS); and ages at follow-up were 10 to 16 years (mean 13 years) (NS). Initial economic classes were 3.4, 3.3, and 3.4 respectively (NS). At initial evaluation the children in the methylphenidate group were less active (Werry Weiss Peters Scale) and had better families than those in the other two groups, but had worse Bender-Gestalt evaluations, indicating the difficulty in matching children perfectly in groups.

Follow-up evaluation measures were:

1. Changes in hyperactivity scores, by the Werry Weiss Peters Scale
2. Assessment of emotional adjustment based on a three-point scale on seven subitems:
   a. peer relations
   b. mood

   c. sexual adjustment
   d. relationship with adults
   e. adjustment to authority
   f. total number of complaints
   g. number of nervous symptoms, (e.g., tics, phobias)
3. Ratings of antisocial behavior on a three-point scale
4. Family Rating Scale at initial and at follow-up evaluation, based on six subitems:
   a. mental health of parents
   b. number of moves
   c. marital relationship
   d. continuous presence of mother (or stable mother substitute)
   e. deviant child rearing practices
   f. level of anxiety present in family interactions
5. Assessment of mother-child relationship on a five-point scale
6. Mother's impression of change (or improvement) in past five years
7. Wechsler Intelligence Scale for Children (WISC), at initial and follow-up evaluation
8. Bender-Gestalt at initial and follow-up evaluation
9. Number of school grades failed
10. Report cards
11. Teacher ratings of conduct

Results indicated that there were no differences between the groups as to IQ, WISC changes, changes on the Bender-Gestalt, changes in family functioning, or in the degree of reduction of hyperactivity ratings. (All three groups scored lower on the hyperactivity scale 5 years later.) On the three measures which were rated at 5-year follow-up only, namely, emotional adjustment, antisocial behavior, and mother's impression of change, no differences were found between the three groups.

With respect to academic performance, there was a trend for the children in the methylphenidate-treated group to have failed fewer grades.

The 12 children who were still receiving methylphenidate at the time of the 5-year follow-up evaluation were taken off the drug 2 weeks prior to testing. As a result their behavior worsened both at home and at school.

With respect to prognostic indicators in all three groups, the initial full-scale WISC correlated significantly with school performance. Initial ratings of hyperactivity had a variable and unpredictable relation to outcome measures. The family rating scale failed to predict outcome on any measures in the chlorpromazine and no-drug groups, but in the methylphenidate-treated group a "good" family correlated significantly with a favorable outcome as measured by academic achievement, abatement of antisocial behavior and emotional adjustment.

Conclusions

1. For all the 12 children still taking methylphenidate at 5-year follow-up, discontinuing the drug produced worsening of behavior at home and at school, indicating that the drug was still of benefit.

2. Outcome measures such as antisocial behavior, emotional adjustment, and degree of improvement noted by mother, did not favor the methylphenidate-treated group.

3. There was a trend for the children treated with methylphenidate to have failed fewer grades.

4. Only in the methylphenidate group was there a significant interaction between a good family and outcome measures, indicating that there is an interaction between a useful drug and a good family that favorably influences prognosis.

Criticisms of the Study

1. Were the measures of outcome too insensitive? For example, no measures of self-esteem were included nor could we assess the degree to which life had become easier on siblings and parents.

2. Were the three groups comparable? They were not randomly assigned in the first place. Both the chlorpromazine-treated group and the stimulant-treated group represented a selection of children from initial drug studies (one in 1964 and 1967 respectively) who had remained on the drug rather than discontinuing it. Children who remain longer on a medication do so because their problems are severe enough to warrant use of the drug and because they are responders. The no-drug group represented parents who did not wish their children to remain on drugs in spite of severe symptoms.

3. The children in the no-drug group and those in the chlorpromazine group were initially assessed and their 5-year outcomes were evaluated 4 years before the initial assessment and 5-year outcome evaluation of the methylphenidate group. This was an advantage in that the no-drug group had never been offered stimulants (because we were not using stimulants from 1962 to 1966), but it was an obvious disadvantage for increasing errors of measurement.

4. The stimulant-treated group was composed of 24 children, of an initial 50 children, all of whom received methylphenidate in an acute drug trial. Ten of the 50 were not followed. Two were eliminated from the study for matching purposes. Eighteen did not remain on methylphenidate for long enough periods to qualify to be in the methylphenidate group. There were no differences on any initial evaluation measures between the 26 treated for at least 3 years and the 18 treated for a shorter period. Ten of the 18 children were non-responders and took methylphenidate for only 1–3 months. Eight children took methylphenidate for up to 3 years. These were not included in the methylphenidate group and could have biased the results obtained, although the direction of bias is not clear in that there was no difference on any measure at the initial assessment.

If it is correct that hyperactive children who are treated longer with any drug are a selected group of more severely disabled children, this would tend to discriminate against the methylphenidate and chlorpromazine groups. There is, however, no evidence that this bias would discriminate more against the methylphenidate than the chlorpromazine group.

5. Not all children began medication, as suggested, in the first grade. In addition, outcome was assessed in adolescence.

"A Two-year Follow-up of 72 Hyperactive Boys: Classroom Behaviour and Peer Acceptance"[18,19]

In a previous publication these authors reported on a 1-year follow-up of the 76 hyperactive middle-class boys, all of whom had participated in a comparative study of methylphenidate, imipramine, and placebo.[19] Children from disturbed homes were not included in the study. A matched control group of 12 children, who had initially responded to the active drug but whose parents had nevertheless discontinued medication within 4 months, served as a control group. Outcome measures used were Conners Teacher's Rating Scale (TRS), Conners Parent Symptom Questionnaire (PSQ), WISC, Wide Range Achievement Test (WRAT), Porteus Maze, and the author's own global rating scale. Results indicated that at 1 year there were no differences between the children on active drugs (methylphenidate and imipramine) and those on no drugs on the PSQ scale, on which all children had improved equally. However, on the 16 Teacher's Rating Scales only the children on active drugs had improved.

Seventy-two of the 76 hyperactive middle-class children were followed for a second year. The initial hyperactive control group of children (who had been active responders but who had discontinued using the drug within 4 months) was, unfortunately, not included in the 2-year follow-up study. Instead, a matched control group of normal children was obtained. The mean age of the children at 2-year follow-up was 10.2 years. Forty-seven of 72 boys (65 percent) were still on methylphenidate (40) or imipramine (7). More than half of the total sample had had either psychiatric treatment or remedial education, with 16 of 72 boys having been referred for long-term psychiatric treatment.

Only 2 of 72 parents stated that they had no serious concern about their son. Sixty-five percent of the parents stated that impulsivity and/or immaturity was their chief concern, while 30% were most concerned with academic difficulties. Three children had had court contact for setting fires or causing injury to other children, and two had threatened sexual molestation. Fifteen hyperactive children had repeated one grade or more and 14 had been placed in special classes.

Selected Thematic Apperception Test (TAT) cards analyzed for depression showed that the hyperactive children were significantly more depressed than the normal controls. The hyperactive group performed significantly worse than normal controls on the Wide Range Achievement Tests (WRAT). The WRAT reading scores at 2 years did not show change over 2 years, while WRAT maths scores for the hyperactive group decreased over 2 years. The WRAT scores of 20 children who had been on continuous treatment with methylphenidate were identical to the test scores of the whole hyperactive sample. Both parents' and teachers' ratings of peer acceptance indicated considerably less social success for hyperactive boys as compared with matched normal controls. Restlessness and conduct disturbances (from teachers' and parents' rating scales) showed improvement at 2-year follow-up, but where significantly higher than for normal control children.

The conclusions reached by the authors were as follows: "This 2-year follow-up study of a relatively homogeneous 'optimally treated' population of hyperactive boys indicates that, as in other studies, this group is at high risk for continuing academic and social difficulty. As 55% of the group were still receiving a stimulant and 9% were taking tricyclic antidepressants after 2 years and a large number also had other academic and psychiatric aid, this outcome is disappointing." This study provides indirect support for the idea that the medication's long-term effect is mainly suppression of impulsive and hyperactive behavior.

Conclusions

It seems that as a result of the beneficial reports from acute drug studies with stimulants for hyperactive children, too much is expected from their long-term use. It has been found that the stimulants have a valuable long-term symptom suppressant effect, but that hyperactive children who take them generally continue to have academic and social problems. Interventions aimed directly toward the amelioration of academic and social interactional problems of these children are obviously required as well as or instead of medication, depending on the needs of the individual child. Studies of hyperactive children as young adults[20] have indicated that many of the earlier problems are eventually outgrown and that the remaining problems center around self-esteem and impulsivity. Whatever can be done in childhood to prevent loss of self-esteem and better socialization skills will be of great value to the final outcome.

References

1. Bradley, C.: The behavior of children receiving benzedrine. *Am J Psychiatry* **94:** 557, 1937.
2. Winsberg, B., Bialer, I., Kupietz, S., and Tobias, J.: Effects of imipramine and dextroamphetamine on behavior of neuropsychiatrically impaired children. *Am J Psychiatry* **128:** 109–115, 1972.
3. Conners, C.K., and Eisenberg, L.: The effects of methylphenidate on symptomatology and learning in disturbed children. *Am J Psychiatry* **120:** 458, 1963.
4. Conners, C.K., Eisenberg, L., and Barcai, A.: Effect of dextroamphetamine on children: Studies on subjects with learning disabilities and school behavior problems. *Arch Gen Psychiatry* **17:** 478, 1967.
5. Weiss, G., Minde, K., Douglas V., et al: Comparison of the effects of chlorpromazine, dextroamphetamine and methylphenidate on the behavior and intellectual functioning of hyperactive children. *Can Med Assoc J* **104:** 20, 1971.
6. Denhoff, E., Davis, A., and Hawkins, R.: Effect of dextroamphetamine on hyperkinetic children: A controlled double blind study. *J Learn Disabil* **4:** 27, 1971.
7. Conners, C.K., and Rothchild, G.: Drugs and learning in children. In *Learning Disorders*, Vol. 3, J. Helmut, Ed. Seattle, Spec. Child, 1968, pp. 193–223.
8. Sykes, D.H., Douglas, V.I., and Morgenstern, G.: The effect of methylphenidate (Ritalin) on sustained attention in hyperactive children. *Psychopharmacologia* **25:** 262, 1972.
9. Conners, C.K., Eisenberg, L., and Sharpe, L.: Effect of methylphenidate (Ritalin) on paired associate learning and Porteus maze performance in emotionally disturbed children. *J Consult Psychol* **28:** 14, 1964.
10. Sprague, R.L., Barnes, K.R., and Werry, J.S.: Methylphenidate and thioridazine: Learning reaction time, activity, and classroom behavior in emotionally disturbed children. *Am J Orthopsychiatry* **40:** 615, 1970.
11. Knights, R.M., and Hinton, G.G.: The effects of methylphenidate (Ritalin) on the motor skills and behavior of children with learning problems. *J Nerv Ment Dis* **148:** 643, 1969.

12. Campbell, S., Douglas, V.I., and Morgenstem, G.: Cognitive styles in hyperactive children and the effect of methylphenidate. *J Child Psychol Psychiatry* **12:** 55, 1971.
13. Mendelson, W., Johnson, N., and Stewart, M.: Hyperactive children as teenagers: A follow-up study. *J Nerv Ment Dis* **153:** 273–279, 1971.
14. Weiss, G., Minde, K., Werry, J.S., et al: Studies on the hyperactive child: Five year follow-up. *Arch Gen Psychiatry* **24:** 409–414, 1971.
15. Minde, K., Weiss, G., and Mendelson, N.: A five year follow-up study of 91 hyperactive school children. *J Am Acad Child Psychiatry* **11:** 595–610, 1972.
16. Sleator, E.K., Neumann, A., and Sprague, R.L.: Hyperactive children: A continuous long term placebo controlled follow-up. *JAMA* **229:** 316–317, 1974.
17. Weiss, G., Kruger, E., Danielson, V., and Elman, M.: Effect of long term treatment of hyperactive children with methylphenidate. *Can Med Assoc J* **112:** 159, 1975.
18. Riddle, K.D., and Rapoport, J.L.: A 2-year follow-up of 72 hyperactive boys. *J Nerv Ment Dis* **162:** 126–134, 1976.
19. Quinn, P.O., and Rapoport, J.L.: One year follow-up of hyperactive boys treated with Imipramine or Methylphenidate. *Am J Psychiatry* **132:** 241–245, 1975.
20. Hechtman, L., Weiss, G., Finklestein, J., Wener, A., and Benn, R.: Hyperactives as young adults: Preliminary report. *Can Med Assoc J* **115:** 625, 1976.

Appendix

WERRY-WEISS-PETERS ACTIVITY SCALE

	NO	*YES—A LITTLE BIT*	*YES—VERY MUCH*
DURING MEALS			
Up and down at table	☐	☐	☐
Interrupts without regard	☐	☐	☐
Wriggling	☐	☐	☐
Fiddles with things	☐	☐	☐
Talks excessively	☐	☐	☐
TELEVISION			
Gets up and down during program	☐	☐	☐
Wriggles	☐	☐	☐
Manipulates objects or body	☐	☐	☐
Talks incessantly	☐	☐	☐
Interrupts	☐	☐	☐
DOING HOME-WORK			
Gets up and down	☐	☐	☐
Wriggles	☐	☐	☐
Manipulates objects or body	☐	☐	☐
Talks incessantly	☐	☐	☐
Requires adult supervision or attendance	☐	☐	☐
PLAY			
Inability for quiet play	☐	☐	☐
Constantly changing activity	☐	☐	☐
Seeks parental attention	☐	☐	☐
Talks excessively	☐	☐	☐
Disrupts other's play	☐	☐	☐

	NO	*YES—A LITTLE BIT*	*YES—VERY MUCH*
SLEEP			
Difficulty settling down for sleep	☐	☐	☐
Inadequate amount of sleep	☐	☐	☐
Restless during sleep	☐	☐	☐
BEHAVIOR AWAY FROM HOME (except School)			
Restlessness during travel	☐	☐	☐
Restlessness during shopping (includes touching everything)	☐	☐	☐
Restlessness during church/movies	☐	☐	☐
Restlessness during visiting friends, relatives, etc.	☐	☐	☐
SCHOOL BEHAVIOR			
Up and down	☐	☐	☐
Fidgets, wriggles, touches	☐	☐	☐
Interrupts teacher or other children excessively	☐	☐	☐
Constantly seeks teacher's attention	☐	☐	☐
TOTAL SCORE	____	____	____

9

Hyperkinesis in Mental Retardation

Siegfried Pueschel, M.D.

Hyperkinesis in Mental Retardation

The observation that mentally retarded children often exhibit hyperkinetic behavior poses a number of relevant questions:

Do retarded children with hyperkinesis differ from those hyperactive children with average intelligence? And if we should find that the retarded child is at variance, in what way is he dissimilar from the nonretarded child with hyperkinesis? Does his neurophysiological function differ significantly when compared with the intellectually normal hyperkinetic child? Is there a distinguishable neurochemical disturbance present in the hyperactive retarded youngster? Does the mentally handicapped child respond differently to therapy in comparison to the "normal" child?

Our experience in the Child Development Center during the past decade revealed that hyperkinesis differs very little in the mentally retarded child when compared with the normal child. In the

Associate Professor of Pediatrics, Section of Reproductive and Developmental Medicine, Brown University, Providence, Rhode Island.
Director, Child Development Center, Rhode Island Hospital, Providence, Rhode Island.

retarded youngster the motor activity is also far in excess of the normal range for age, sex, and environment. The hyperactive child with mental retardation also has boundless energy; he is on the go all the time, he shifts from one activity to another. He has poor judgment, limited attention span, is easily distracible and often needs constant supervision. His overactivity, irritability, and erratic behavior exhaust parents and teachers alike.

Most families can deal with and adjust to the retardation aspect, but what is so frustrating to parents and siblings and drives friends out of the house is that the child is on the move 24 hours a day, and his purposeless constant activity and decreased emotional stability interfere with normal family life. Because of his retardation, the parents say that they cannot "get through to him." The teachers likewise are at their wits' end since the difficulties in providing an appropriate educational experience for the mentally handicapped youngster is compounded by his inability to concentrate, to sit still, and to pay attention.

The only rational approach to the problem at hand is comprehensive management. This should begin with a thorough multidisciplinary evaluation of the child in order to identify his weaknesses and strengths. This evaluation should involve a social service interview to shed light on the family dynamics; psychological and educational assessments to determine the child's cognitive abilities and academic capabilities so important for subsequent educational recommendations. Other disciplines including child psychiatry, neurology, and a speech and language evaluation also contribute to the comprehensive evaluation of the child.

Based on this assessment, recommendations for total management can then be formulated. Central nervous system stimulating drugs may be a welcome adjunct (if the child responds appropriately) since this might permit him to settle down, to concentrate, and to pay attention. Thus, he might be able to participate in a meaningful learning experience. Specified supportive education tailored to the individual child's need should be forthcoming in an environment void of too many distractions.

Often the parents will be in need of counseling. They will have to learn to understand their child's actions and reactions in order to assist in the treatment program. The difficulties in explaining the medical aspects to the parents so that they can understand the situation is a reflection of the problem the medical community itself has in understanding this syndrome complex. By helping the parents comprehend that their child's behavior pattern is not a result of parental mismanagement but rather stems from difficulties in neurophysiological control mechanisms in the child, the physician will relieve some of the feelings of confusion, guilt, and hostility which often accompany the parent–child relationship. The child should also be told that he does have a problem, but that it did not occur through any fault of his own and that various things can and will be done to help him. To deny any problems or to avoid talking about them may result in the child thinking that he has a far worse illness or condition perhaps one too terrible to even talk about.

The home environment may need adjustment. Siblings at times will have to be involved in the management program, and parents are in need of supportive guidance in consistent behavior management of their child. Behavior therapy in school in the form of operant conditioning with carry over into the home situation has been shown to benefit not only the child but the entire family.

Recreational activities which should be enjoyed by all family members will often provide "outlets" to channel the overactivity into fun-type games. After-school programs, weekend scouting, and summertime camp experiences are but a few areas where the hyperactive retarded child will find the needed recreation. These time periods when the child is out of the home will then allow the parents to unwind and to relax. It is of paramount importance to realize that the problem of the hyperkinetic child affects every aspect of his family's daily life. Continued warm and friendly concern on the part of the involved professional will provide the needed emotional support to the family. His active involvement will tell the family that he cares, and this will make a significant impact on the future of this child.

A number of syndromes have been described in the literature on hyperactivity and mental retardation. In this presentation we will focus on two more common disease entities where hyperkinesis has been observed.

When we were involved in the lead poisoning screening study in the Roxbury section of Boston,[9] we saw many children with an increased lead burden who displayed symptoms usually observed in the hyperkinetic impulse disorder as defined by Dr. Denhoff. Those children had reportedly a short attention span; they shifted from one activity to another; they showed an excessive activity level being in constant motion; and they exhibited impulsiveness and an inability to delay gratification. When compared with a matched control population without lead poisoning, there was a significant excess of children with hyperkinetic behavior in the study group.[6]

Such observations were also reported by other investigators.

David presented a paper at a lead poisoning conference in North Carolina on the association between lead poisoning and hyperactivity. He looked at his population from a different point of view, comparing hyperactive children with a normal active control group. He found that the hyperactive children had significantly higher blood lead levels, increased postpencillamine urine lead levels, and more frequent lead exposure.[3] Baloh and his group noted similar findings when they studied neuropsychological effects of chronic lead absorption.[2] In the subjects with increased lead levels, there was a significantly increased incidence of hyperkinetic behavior.

It should be emphasized that not all children with lead poisoning are mentally retarded. On the contrary, the majority of children with an increased lead burden in our study were in the low average range of intellectual functioning. Yet a somewhat higher percentage of retarded children exhibited hyperkinesis.[7]

An elegant study was carried out by Allen and co-workers focusing on the pathobiological and behavioral effects of lead intoxication in the infant Rhesus monkey. They observed altered social interaction, tremors, and hyperactivity after lead intoxication.[1]

In their animal experiments, Silbergeld and Goldberg found that excessive lead exposure in food caused an increased activity level which was three times as high as in age-matched controls.[10] Interestingly, the lead-treated animals responded paradoxically to amphetamines and methylphenidate; i.e., the central nervous system stimulants suppressed their hyperactivity while phenobarbital exacerbated the lead-induced hyperkinesis.

Another mental retardation disorder where hyperkinesis is frequently seen is phenylketonuria (PKU). We have observed in many untreated older patients with PKU, hyperactive behavior, in particular increased repetitive, purposeless movements of the distal extremities. Increased motor activity has also been noted in PKU patients whose phenylalanine-restricted diet had been discontinued and who were eating a regular diet. Irritability and hyperactivity became more pronounced in those patients after a high protein intake.[8]

It is of interest that in the central nervous system, phenylalanine is decarboxylated to phenethylamine, a compound which has amphetamine-like pharmacological properties. Phenethylamine has been found in increased concentrations in brain tissue of untreated PKU patients.[5]

McKean investigated the effects of a high phenylalanine concentration on serotonin and catecholamine metabolism in the human brain. He reported profound disturbance in cerebral serotonin and catecholamine metabolism with associated high plasma concentration of phenylalanine. He could reverse these amine effects in PKU subjects by restricting their phenylalanine intake.[4]

Lead poisoning and phenylketonuria are but two examples where metabolic interference in neurophysiological mechanisms may lead to increased activity in the child. Further investigations in such mental retardation syndromes might bring about a better understanding of the pathogenesis of hyperkinesis in mental retardation.

References

1. Allen, J.R., McWey, P.J., and Suomi, S.J.: Pathobiological and behavioral effects of lead intoxication in the infant rhesus monkey. *Environ Health* Perspect **7:** 239–246, 1974.
2. Baloh, R., Sturm, R., Green, B., and Gleser, G.: Neuropsychological effects of chronic asymptomatic increased lead absorption. *Arch Neurol* **32:** 326–330, 1975.
3. David, O.J.: Association between lower level lead concentrations and hyperactivity in children. *Environ Health Perspect* **7:** 17–25, 1974.
4. McKean, C.M.: The effects of high phenylalanine concentrations on serotonin and catecholamine metabolism in the human brain. *Brain Res.* **47:** 469–476, 1972.
5. Oates, J.A., Nirenberg, P.Z., Jepson, J.B., Sjoerdsma, A., and Udenfriend, S.: Conversion of phenylalanine to phenethylamine in patients with phenylketonuria. *Soc Proc Exp Biol Med* **112:** 1078–1081, 1963.
6. Pueschel, S.M.: Neurological and psychomotor functions in children with an increased lead burden. *Environ Health Perspect* **4:** 13–16, 1974.
7. Pueschel, S.M.: Unpublished data.
8. Pueschel, S.M.: Unpublished data.
9. Pueschel, S.M., Kopito, L., and Schwachman, H.: Children with an increased lead burden. *JAMA* **222:** 462–466, 1972.
10. Silbergeld, E.K., and Goldberg, A.M.: Hyperactivity: A lead-induced behavior disorder. *Environ Health Perspect* **7:** 227–232, 1974.

10

Minimal Brain Dysfunction: Factors Leading to Breakdown in Adulthood

Allan Berman, Ph.D.

Minimal brain dysfunction has been studied in young children, but there have been few systematic studies of the phenomenon in adolescents and adults. Some investigators have believed that the disorder became less of a problem as the child matured, and even that it disappeared entirely by the onset of puberty. However, very often MBD does not fade away. Moreover, the *effects* of MBD in childhood can set into motion a series of behavioral adjustments that have a significant adverse effect on the behavior of the child and as he grows into adolescence and adulthood.

There are two problems we see in adolescence and adulthood: (1) that of the adult with MBD who may still need medical treatment, and (2) that of the adult in whom the behavioral consequences of MBD have shaped a life-style that may no longer be conducive to adjustment. While the incidence of MBD among adolescents and adults is still being debated, very few of those professionals involved with the problem deny that the behavioral consequences of years of childhood MBD can create patterns of reactions that may lead to disturbances or failure to cope after childhood.

Professor of Psychology, Department of Psychology, University of Rhode Island, Kingston, Rhode Island.

Research on the etiology of delinquency has resulted in interesting implications for the study of MBD. The results suggested that we can predict, from family and school adjustment patterns, which MBD or MBD-like children are most likely to be high risk for acting-out or delinquency behaviors as adolescents.

The research was done at the Rhode Island Training Schools and at Central High School in Providence. Grim statistics provide stark evidence of the failure of most current and traditional rehabilitation programs for delinquents. Despite all the funds and professional time that has been devoted to the study of delinquency over the past two decades, the rate of delinquency continues to climb, as does the rate of recidivism, and the mean age at which a child first becomes delinquent is decreasing. Thus, children now are likely to first become delinquent at the age of 12 or 13, and 75–80% of these children will be in and out of reformatories and prisons for the rest of their lives. In addition, dropout rates in high schools are increasing, and one out of every three youngsters who drops out of school before age 16 will become adjudicated as delinquent.[6]

Psychodynamic and psychosocial explanations and treatments of delinquency have not been successful in reducing the incidence of these cases. In trying to develop alternative approaches, we observed the youth carefully. We noticed that most of the delinquent teenagers we worked with were very poorly skilled in a number of basic daily living tasks. Rather than exhibiting traditional signs of psychopathology, they showed evidence of inadequate coping and learning skills. They were poorly coordinated, seemed to have problems understanding things, and had obviously inadequate academic skills. Using a comprehensive battery of neuropsychological tests, we sought to determine what levels of skill these youngsters had, and in what skillls they were deficient.

We examined 122 delinquents and 45 comparison youngsters of equivalent age and grade level, who were still in high school and never had exhibited any delinquent behavior. All youngsters in both groups were given the Halstead-Reitan Neuropsychology Battery, along with the Wechsler Intelligence Test, a detailed interview and history, academic achievement tests, and a few other diagnostic tests used for their interpretive value.

The criteria used were the standardized cutoff scores for each Halstead-Reitan subtest. Each subject was scored as either in the normal or the impaired range on each Halstead-Reitan test. A subject was considered dysfunctional if he scored in the impaired range on at least one of the Halstead-Reitan tests. No subject was classified as impaired based on any of the other test results or other data that were accumulated.

We found that 70% of the delinquent group showed impairment on at least one Halstead-Reitan test, and 56% showed impairment on at least two subtests. In the comparison group, 23% showed at least one impairment. In addition, due to the sophistication of the Halstead-Reitan Battery for neuropsychological diagnosis, a complicated system of four simultaneous methods of scoring can be used to determine indicators of chronicity as well as the likely etiology of the disorder. We did those calculations and, in addition, accumulated historical and behavioral data which allowed us to make confident conclusions about etiology.

There are several levels to the conclusions which can be made. First, and most clearly, 70% of the delinquents were clearly impaired in one or more important skills necessary for competence both in school and in routine adjustment to the environment. The types of skills they were lacking are familiar to us: visual/perceptual dysfunction, auditory memory disorder, and nonverbal concept formation were the most common deficits in our group. In addition, there were auditory discrimination deficits, visual-sequential disorders, and inefficiencies in tactile/kinesthetic feedback. All of these dysfunctions appeared a significant number of times, and with more frequency in the delinquent group than in the comparison group. These dysfunctions are similar to those which appear in young children with learning disabilities or MBD.

This study[3,4] as well as earlier projections of the data[1,2] documented specifically the relationship between learning disabilities and juvenile delinquency. The evidence is now so convincing that the National Council of Juvenile Court Judges includes a training session in learning disabilities in all its training colleges for new judges, and the Federal government has proposed new regulations to include learning disabilitiy as a handicap worthy of special assistance. The Law Enforcement Assistance Administration has also recently allotted over 1½ million dollars in grants to Creighton University and the National Association for Children with Learning Disabilities to study the relationship between delinquency and learning disabilities and recommend appropriate treatments.

Simply showing a relationship between learning disabilities and delinquency is not sufficient. We need to know if the learning disabilities caused the delinquency or whether it was a significant causative factor. We also need to know whether MBD was originally (or whether it continues to be) the cause of the disabilities. While the data are still speculative, there are several pieces of evidence which do support the notion that significant numbers of delinquents now have, or once had, MBD, and that the MBD or associated learning disabilities played a significant role in the development of the delinquent life-style.

I will briefly summarize these pieces of evidence:

1. A consulting neurologist was brought in from another state to provide independent validation of our diagnoses. Unfamiliar with the hypotheses of the study, the neurologist was presented with 42 subjects and asked to perform a neurologic examination and provide a diagnosis. Of the 42 subjects, 30 were considered impaired on the basis of our testing and 12 were normal. The neurologist was not told which group was which, nor the numbers of each in the sample. None of the 12 normals was diagnosed as impaired by the neurologist. Of the 30 youngsters in our impaired group, the neurologist found impairment in 27 (90% agreement). While specific diagnoses varied, all impaired subjects were diagnosed as having some type of chronic, static disorder, and most frequently (16 of 27) the diagnosis included the phrase "most consistent with a chronic, diffuse, minimal or nonspecific neurological disorder." When discussing his evaluations with us later, after he had been informed of the purposes of the study, the neurologist agreed that our subjects most likely had been impaired since early childhood, and that the most appropriate of the common diagnostic categories to describe them would be MBD.

2. A study of the available school and behavorial records, as well as the detailed histories of our subjects, revealed that most had been in continual academic and learning distress since the early school years. Their records were filled not only with evidence of learning disorders and failures, but also with comments of teachers and school consultants regarding their behavior. As far as can be determined by this type of retrospective data, if appropriate professional help had been available, we are confident that these youngsters would have been diagnosed as having MBD. Significantly, none of them had been diagnosed, either as having MBD or as being learning disabled.

3. Useful information, as well as perplexing questions, are derived from comparing results between our delinquent group and the comparison group. Keep in mind that the comparison group was very carefully selected to be matched controls for the group in the training schools. They were equivalent in terms of socioeconomic background, educational level (in terms of achievement test scores), age, race, and sex. Moreover, interviews with family as well as school personnel convinced us that our comparison subjects were free of

behaviors that might be considered delinquent. We had a comparison group that was similar in most respects to the delinquent group, except that the comparison group members had never been delinquent or engaged in known criminal behaviors.

It is the very closeness of the comparison that provides us with the questions. As mentioned above 23% of this comparison group showed disabilities similar to those in the delinquent group. While this is a reasonable figure in terms of the percentages of disabled children found in many school systems, we have to ask why the 23%, so similar to the delinquents, managed to avoid delinquency. If they came from the same types of socioeconomic backgrounds, had similar other characteristics as our delinquents, and also had early disabilities, why hadn't they also become delinquent? How did they make it successfully?

One obvious clue is in the various school and historical records we examined. While we observed the same learning problems reported above for the delinquents, there were two differences in the backgrounds of the nondelinquents, differences which may be important: (1) *most of this 23% group had been diagnosed as learning disabled or as having MBD*, whereas none of the delinquents had been; and (2) we did not find in their records nearly as much incidence of behavioral acting-out problems in school as in the delinquents.

These pieces of evidence, albeit circumstantial, provide a strong argument that, among the delinquents in our sample who showed significant disabilities, most if not all had been disabled, probably from MBD, since early childhood. The fact that they were not properly diagnosed and treated set into motion a devastating series of events that, for a large number, resulted in a delinquent life-style.

There are three basic reasons why the delinquents became delinquent:

1. *Undiagnosed and untreated MBD and/or learning disabilities in childhood.* This seems to be a pivotal factor, since 70% of the delinquent group showed these problems. The critical words here are *undiagnosed* and *untreated*, since the incidence of later delinquency drops sharply if the MBD or disabilities are properly diagnosed and treated.

2. *Continual failure in school*, moreover failure that is assumed by parents, teachers, and professionals to be due to lack of motivation by the child, rather than to the child's inability to function.

3. *Nonsupportive family situation.* The use of this term is to distinguish what is meant from the usual terminology about family intactness. It refers not to whether the family is "broken" or has certain people living in it, but simply to whether the family, or

anyone in it, supports the child when the school problems begin. Does the family sympathize with the child and try to build up his self-esteem in the face of continual failure, or does the family support the school's mistaken approach to the child's problems, making the child feel inadequate?

It should be noted that these results suggest strongly that socioeconomic status, a frequently alleged cause of delinquency, is not a primary factor. Our results suggest that the most serious effect of socioeconomic status is that children from lower socioeconomic families are at a somewhat higher risk of having their disorders go undetected. Insofar as we can determine, however, the old assumptions that socioeconomic problems are at the root of delinquency are as unfounded as the psychodynamic assumptions about delinquency—neither assumption has produced any programs that have been effective in keeping youngsters from turning in increasing numbers to delinquency.

The cycle begins at home, and is reinforced by poor school methods. Usually the child shows attentional or perceptual problems even before starting school, but this behavior is dismissed as ornery or uncooperative. The child enters the early years of school already feeling that he often cannot do things right, and that new tasks will mean humiliation and failure. This prophecy becomes fulfilled when teachers punish and ridicule the child for learning and behavior problems he cannot control. The child develops the self-image of a loser, as someone who can never hope to live up to what people expect of him.

At about the third grade, the first of a series of crucial happenings that differentiate future delinquents from nondelinquents can be noted. If the impaired child gets through the third grade without significant failure or humiliating experiences, the chances are excellent that he has a fairly supportive home and will continue to get by in school. However, children from nonsupportive homes, during the third grade, show a characteristic change in their peer group preferences. Rather than associating with the youngsters who live near them or who sit near them at school, they withdraw from their customary friendships and move toward alliances with other children in the class who have become school problems, for whatever reason. This seemingly simple event, often barely noticeable at the time, occurs with great reliability during the third grade or early fourth grade, and has been shown to be related to non-supportive homes as well as to later incidences of delinquency.

Then we see the behavioral signs become more pronounced than the original learning problems. Clowning around and general disruptiveness become the youngster's best insulation against having to face continual failure and frustration. He becomes more successful and respected by peers as a troublemaker than he ever was as a student. Teachers are now solely diverted from the learning problems and concentrate almost exclusively on how to control behavior. The problems become more severe; by the fifth or sixth grade the child is either being suspended regularly or not going to school. Attendance is irregular, and the stage has been set for dropping out and eventual delinquency.

Once this cycle begins it is vicious and insidious. Our study in Rhode Island, as well as a study with a larger sample in Colorado,[5] have demonstrated that 75–80% of delinquents can be shown to follow this pattern, which has only recently become discernible. The record is all the more discouraging since *at no point in this destructive cycle has the basic impairment been realized or addressed.*

This research has resurrected a way of understanding some problems of adolescence and young adulthood that reminds us of earlier approaches that emphasized physiologic rather than psychological causality. While we have no evidence or belief that there is a physiological cause of delinquency, we feel that we have sufficient data to suggest that undiagnosed, untreated MBD or learning disabilities can be shown to begin a specific, destructive series of behavioral and environmental events which results in many children ending up on the wrong side of the courts. It is clear that more sufficient longitudinal and etiologic studies must be done to verify some of the suggestions made here. However, it is also clear that the effects of untreated or poorly treated MBD can be quite severe as the child matures. Anyone who questions the need for studying and further understanding MBD need only look at what happens to young people in whom the problem is ignored.

References

1. Berman, A.: Learning disabilities in juvenile delinquents. Presented to the Seventh Annual Spring Conference of the Massachusetts Association for Children with Learning Disabilities. Boston, Massachusetts, 1973.
2. Berman, A.: Delinquents are disabled. In *Youth In Trouble*, B. Kratoville, Ed. Academic Therapy Press, New York, 1974.
3. Berman, A., and Siegal, A.: Adaptive and learning skills in juvenile delinquents—A neuropsychological analysis. *J Learn Disabil* **9:** 583–590, 1976a.
4. Berman, A., and Siegal, A.: A neuropsychological approach to the etiology, prevention and treatment of juvenile delinquency. In *Child Personality and Psychopathology, Current Topics, Vol. III*, A. Davids, Ed. Wiley, New York, 1976b.
5. Compton, R.: A plan for skill deficit training at Lathrop Park Youth Camp. In *Youth In Trouble, op. cit.*, 1974.
6. Poremba, C.: Learning disabilities among delinquents. Presented at the Annual Meeting of the International Association for Children with Learning Disabilities, Houston, Texas, 1975.

11

The Attention Disorders and Related Syndromes: Outcome in Adolescence and Young Adult Life

Steven A. Feldman, M.D., Eric Denhoff, M.D.,
and Joseph I. Denhoff, M.S.

There are conflicting reports in the literature as to the status in adolescence and adulthood of children earlier diagnosed as having minimal brain dysfunction (MBD) or the hyperkinetic impulse disorder (HID),* now collectively called the attentional disorders.[1–4] This is a report of an investigation of the later outcome of such individuals.

All the children in this study had been referred to a practice-oriented multidisciplinary group for the diagnosis and treatment of

Governor Medical Center, and the Departments of Pediatrics and Psychiatry, Brown University, Providence, Rhode Island.

* The hyperkinetic impulse disorder (as defined by Laufer and Denhoff[5]) is characterized by hyperactivity, short attention span, and poor powers of concentration (particularly under school conditions), as well as variability, explosive irritability, and low frustration tolerance.

The minimal brain dysfunction syndrome includes children who are hyperkinetic in addition to those children of near average, average, or above-average intelligence who have deviations of central nervous system function manifested by various combinations of impairments in perception, conceptualization, language, and memory.[6]

learning disorders.** Each had been found to be the result of or associated with an attentional disorder and/or MBD.

Methods

Patients

By means of record review and personal contact, we selected for study and obtained comprehensive evaluations on 81 adolescents and 48 young adult former patients who had either HID or MBD as the basis for their problems.

Selection Criteria

The subjects selected had a full scale IQ score of 80 or higher and no evidence of primary emotional problems, seizure disorders, or cerebral palsy.

Adolescent Group

The 81 adolescents underwent physical and neurologic examinations and an interview, which assessed emotional and sexual adjustment; mood; relationships with parents, peers, and authority figures; and quality of school performance. Particular attention was given to patterns of drug and alcohol use, and to the presence of delinquent behavior. Hyperactivity was rated on the Werry-Weiss-Peters Scale of Hyperactivity.[7]

After being evaluated, the patient was assigned a psychiatric impairment scale rating according to the description of Gross and Wilson.[8] This scale rates impairment from nonexistent (0) through average (3) to severe and requiring institutional treatment (see Appendix).

** The Governor Medical Center and the Governor Center School in Providence, Rhode Island, are staffed by clinical psychologists, special educators, language and visual perception therapists, and psychiatric social workers.

Treatment available at the Center includes medical care and medication, specific visual perceptual remediation, psychotherapy, parental casework, family therapy, school consultation and special education, and speech and language therapy.

In 1973, the Governor Medical Center established a division of Adolescent and Young Adult Medicine, and all patients over the age of 12 years were transferred to the care of the senior author (S.A.F.)

The team leaders responsible for continuity of care as well as the medical aspects and medications were Eric Denhoff, M.D., a specialist in developmental pediatrics, and Maurice W. Laufer, M.D., a child psychiatrist.

Young Adults

The 48 young adults also were evaluated. Each subject had a physical and neurologic examination and filled out the Tennessee Self-Concept Inventory[9] and a questionnaire designed to assess both individual and family drug and alcohol use patterns.[10] Responses were checked by interview. All subjects were given the Slosson Drawing Coordination Test[11] and were tested on items reflecting auditory sequential memory and auditory short-term memory, such as reciting the months of the year in order and repeating a simple sentence.[12]

After these evaluations had been completed, siblings over age 18 of the young adults were mailed the self-concept inventory, the drawing coordination test, and the drug and alcohol questionnaire.[13] Thirty-two siblings participated in this study.

Responses to the drug and alcohol questions were compared with normative data on drug and alcohol use in the State of Rhode Island, which are on file in the Community Medicine Section of Brown University in Providence, Rhode Island.[10,13]

For the Tennessee Self-Concept Inventory, comparisons between the mean responses of the young adults and the siblings were made by means of a *t*-test. Additional *t*-tests were performed to compare the mean responses from each of the groups against the normative values.

The alcohol and drug use questionnaires were analyzed by either the chi-square or the exact probability test.

Results

Adolescents

Eighty-five percent of the youths were male, referred at a mean age of 10 years and reevaluated at a mean of 5½ years later. They had average or better intelligence, and were white middle-class (Table 1).

The most frequent specific diagnoses within the minimal brain dysfunction syndrome included the combination of visual/perceptual/motor difficulties, language impairments, hyperkinetic impulse disorder, and secondary emotional problems in 17 subjects (20%); visual/perceptual/motor, language and hyperkinesis, without secondary emotional problems in 10 subjects (12%); and hyperkinetic impulse disorder alone in 12 subjects (14%) (Table 2).

Causes

Perinatal. The reports of pregnancy and perinatal events were described. In only 15 cases (18%) were there risk factors. Two

TABLE 1
Subjects

	Adolescents	*Young Adults*	*Siblings*
Total	81	48	32
Male	69 (85%)	35 (72%)	15 (46%)
Female	12	13	17
Mean age at Initial Referral (yr)	10 (range, 3 to 16)	9	
Mean age at Current Evaluation (yr)	15.5 (range, 12–20)	21 (range, 18–30)	26
Mean IQ			
WISC Full Scale	99 (range, 80–127)	104 (range, 83–121)	
Verbal	97 (range, 84–126)	105 (range, 84–126)	
Performance	101 (range, 77–127)	(range, 77–127)	
Socioeconomic Status	Middle class (2.9 on modified Hollingshead Scale)		
Race	White	White	White

TABLE 2
Initial Specific Diagnosis in 81 Adolescent Subjects Classified as Having MBD or HID

Dysfunctions				*Number*	*Percent*
VPM[a]	Language	HID	Emotional	17	20
		HID		12	14
VPM	Language	HID		10	12
VPM	Language			9	11
VPM	Language		Emotional	7	8
VPM		HID	Emotional	7	8
		HID	Emotional	5	6
VPM	Language			3	3
VPM			Emotional	3	3
	Language		Emotional	3	3
	Language	HID	Emotional	2	2
	Language	HID		2	2
	Language			1	1

[a] Visual/perceptual/motor.

mothers reported that they were toxemic, and one reported premature placental separation. There were two elective cesarean sections and one breech delivery. One infant sustained a skull fracture during delivery. One infant weighed less than 5 lb (4 lb, 14 oz). One infant required an exchange transfusion, and six mothers reported that their infants required oxygen at birth or during the first few days of life.

Familial or Genetic. Probable emotional, psychiatric, or genetic problems within the family were reported in 26 cases (32%). Ten youths (12%) had been adopted. Eight families had experienced either divorce, separation, or desertion. Significant marital tension was reported in seven families at the time of original diagnosis.

In five families, parental psychiatric difficulties were reported: one father was depressed, and one mother was psychotic. One mother had had a "nervous breakdown," and in one family both parents had had nervous breakdowns. One mother was described as having an "explosive personality."

Eleven families reported difficulties with one or more siblings of the problem child.

In two families, a drinking problem was reported.

Two fathers reported that they had done poorly in school. One father reported an ongoing seizure disorder, while another reported having had seizures in childhood.

Therapy

Eighty-three percent of the subjects received multiple therapy, which often included medication, while medication only was prescribed in 2% (Table 3).

TABLE 3
Treatment

	Adolescent	*Young Adult*
Subjects with Multiple Therapies Including Medication	68/81 (83%)	39/48 (81%)
Subjects with Medication as Sole Therapy	2/81 (2%)	0/48 (0%)
Subjects who received as Components of the Treatment Plan the Following:		
Individual counseling	63/81 (77%)	13/48 (27%)
Family therapy	30/81 (37%)	13/48 (27%)
Visual/perceptual training	28/81 (34%)	12/48 (25%)
Language therapy	23/81 (28%)	3/48 (6%)
Special education	25/81 (30%)	23/48 (47%)

Outcome

In 46 of 81 subjects (57%) there was no evidence to suggest that MBD or HID or its sequelae persisted. In the remaining 35 cases, there was adjustment difficulty and therapeutic intervention was indicated. Of the 35 subjects, 7 (8%) required psychostimulant medication in order to maintain good adjustment patterns and, in one case, both psychostimulant medication and individual counseling were needed. Counseling, usually for self-image, was indicated in 13 cases (16%), and educational modifications were necessary in seven (8%).

Of the 81, 7 youths (8%) had significant problems. Three subjects were drug abusers, three were under the custody of the family court for delinquent behavior, and one girl was a chronic runaway. One of the drug abusers was hospitalized at the State Hospital Adolescent Unit and the runaway was hospitalized at a private psychiatric hospital. All except one of the drug abuse and delinquency cases had had minimal ongoing contact with the Center, because either of the distance involved or poor parental compliance.

In the post-study period, two subjects died of self-inflicted gunshot wounds. One was definitely a suicide; the other may have been accidental (Table 4).

Outcome in Young Adult Life

Characteristics of the 48 young adult males and 32 siblings, representing 19 families, are presented in Table 1.

Most were male, all had average intelligence, or better, and all were white and middle class. The mean age at referral was 9 years

TABLE 4
Outcome in Adolescence

Rating	*Number of Subjects*	*Therapy Needed*	
Good	46/81 (57%)	None	
Fair (Psychiatric Impairment Score 1, 2, 3)	28/81 (35%)	Medication	7/81 (8%)
		Medication and counseling	1/81 (1%)
		Counseling	13/81 (16%)
		Educational modifications	7/81 (8%)
Poor (Score 4, 5, 6)	7/81 (8%)	Family court supervision	3/81 (3%)
		Outpatient drug program	2/81 (2%)
		Inpatient psychiatric care	2/81 (2%)
Fatal[a]	2/81 (2%)		

[a] There were two deaths in the post-study period by self-inflicted gunshot wounds. One was a definite suicide; the other may have been accidental.

and the average age at follow-up was 21 years. Combinations of specific diagnoses similar to those in the adolescent group were found (Table 5). Causes reported by the mother were similar to those in the adolescent group. Six subjects reported that their father had psychiatric problems and six reported that their mother had psychiatric problems. Seven subjects felt that their father had a drinking problem, four felt that their mother had a drinking problem, and two felt that a brother or sister had a drinking problem.

Educational Outcome

Three of the 48 subjects (6%) dropped out of high school or vocational school permanently. The young adult group completed a mean of 13.2 years of schooling as 19 of 48 (39%) went on to higher education. The 32 siblings completed a mean of 14.1 grades.

As in the adolescent group, over 80% received multiple therapy (Table 3). The 32 siblings are described in Table 1.

Self-Concept

A comparison between the mean responses of the young adults diagnosed in childhood as having MBD and their siblings was made for each item in the Tennessee Self-Concept Scale by means of a *t*-test.

Of the results for the Total Self-Concept Score, the most important single score on the scale is presented in Table 6. Those with high scores tended to like themselves, felt they are persons of

TABLE 5
Childhood Diagnosis in 48 Young Adults

Diagnoses				*Number*	*Percent*
VPM[a]		HID		7	14
VPM		HID	Emotional	6	12
		HID	Emotional	6	12
VPM	Language			4	8
VPM			Emotional	4	8
VPM	Language	HID		4	8
	Language		Emotional	4	8
VPM	Language		Emotional	4	8
VPM	Language	HID	Emotional	3	6
	Language			3	6
		HID		2	4
	Language	HID		1	2

[a] Visual/perceptual/motor.

TABLE 6
Results of Statistical Analyses of the Tennessee Self-Concept Scale

Mean Difference	*t*	*p*
Siblings–Young Adults		
29.915	3.236	<0.01
Young Adults–Normals		
−10.80	−2.00	0.05
Siblings–Normals		
15.12	2.62	0.01

worth and value, have confidence in themselves, and act accordingly. Additional *t*-tests were run to compare the mean responses from each group against normative values.

Self-concept ratings for the 48 subjects were within the normal range (30th percentile). For siblings, ratings were significantly higher at the 70th percentile ($p < 0.01$).

Slosson Drawing Coordination Test

Six of 48 subjects (12.5%) failed the test at the eighth through the twelfth grade level. Three of 32 siblings (9%) failed at the same level.

Diadochokinetic Skills

Seven of 48 subjects (14%) had difficulty in performing motor tasks requiring bilateral symmetrical motor organization (diadochokinetic skills).

Auditory Short-Term Memory

Twenty-one of 48 subjects (43%) were unable to pass the test items on the initial try, indicating persistence of inefficient memory, particularly under stress.

Adjustment Patterns

Overall, 44 of 48 subjects (91%) were either in school or working at the time of this evaluation. Significant problems were noted only in 5 of 48 (10%).

One subject was using marijuana daily and had no goals or plans for his future. He had undergone a diagnostic study only at the Center. Another subject, also having had with diagnostic study only, also had no goals and was living at home, not attempting to find a job. Three subjects had severe schizoid personality disturbances—one had been referred to the Center at age 17, one had severe dyslexia and was unable to read, and one had developed severe secondary emotional problems during childhood, which had required 4 years of hospitalization at a children's psychiatric institution.

A higher percentage of the 48 young adults had tried marijuana than the state norms, and fewer had tried barbiturates. The use of psychostimulants was less than in the state generally. Only one subject reported using marijuana daily. There is no evidence that the use of psychostimulant drugs in childhood is associated with drug abuse in young adult life, since there are no statistically significant differences between our study groups and state norms.

Alcohol Use

Brown University studies[10,13] estimate that as many as 15% of students under the age of 25 in Rhode Island may be problem drinkers or potential abusers of alcohol.

Our studies confirmed this finding. Sixteen percent of our 48 young adult subjects reported being drunk before school and 15% reported being drunk more than one time per week. While the abuse of alcohol is cause for concern, there is no evidence that the use of psychostimulant drugs in childhood is associated with increased alcohol problems in young adult life.

Alcohol Questionnaire

Frequency tables of the responses to the alcohol questionnaire are presented in Table 7. In order to test the differences between the young adults and their siblings, with respect to the responses to the items in the questionnaire, either a chi-square test (where appropriate) or an exact probability test was run on each of the tables. The results indicated that the only significant difference was for one item, "drunk before school or work." However, the group differences in the item "frequency of drunkenness," approached a significant level ($p = 0.07$)

Patterns of Nonprescribed Drug Use

The frequency tables of the patterns of nonprescribed drug use are presented in Table 8. The frequencies from a sample of 200

TABLE 7
Results of the Analyses on the Responses to the Alcohol Questionnaire

	Young Adults	Siblings
Frequency of Drunkenness		
At least 3 times per month	13 (27%)	3 (10%)
1–2 times per month	8 (16%)	4 (13%)
1–2 times per year	13 (27%)	12 (40%)
Never Drunk	10 (20%)	11 (36%)
Total	44	30
Chi-square statistic = 5.21		
$p = 0.07$		
Drunk Before School or Work		
Yes	8 (16%)	0
No	40	32
Total	48	32
Exact probability = 0.02		
Have Had a "Blackout"		
Yes	4 (8%)	4 (8%)
No	44	28
Total	48	32
Exact probability = 0.71		
Alcohol Relieves Anxiety, Tension, Depression		
Yes	14 (29%)	7 (21%)
No	34	32
Total	48	32
Chi-square statistic = 0.53		
$p = 0.47$		
Alcohol is a Problem for Subject		
Yes	0	2 (6%)
No	48	30
Total	48	32
Exact probability = 0.16		

people from a normal population are also presented. Because of a small expected cell size, a 2 × 3 chi-square test could not be performed on the item "tried barbiturates," and hence the normal frequencies were not included. For each 2 × 3 table, a chi-square test was run. The results indicate that no significant differences were detected among young adults, siblings, and normals. For the item "tried barbiturates" the exact probability test did not show a significant difference between young adults and siblings.

Discussion

The results reported in this paper suggest that when white middle-class children with MBD or attentional deficits are treated comprehensively in a multidisciplinary setting, the outcome in adolescence and young adult life is favorable. The results also indicate that the use of psychostimulant medications in childhood is not associated

TABLE 8
Results of Analyses on the Patterns of Non-Prescribed Drug Use

	Young Adults	Siblings	Normals
Tried Marijuana			
Yes	24 (50%)	12 (37%)	67 (33%)
No	24	20	133
Total	48	32	200
Chi-square statistic = 4.54			
$p = 0.10$			
Tried Psychedelics			
Yes	7 (14%)	3 (9%)	43 (21%)
No	41	29	157
Total	48	32	200
Chi-square statistic = 3.36			
p = 0.19			
Tried Stimulants			
Yes	10 (20%)	7 (21%)	52 (26%)[a]
No	38	25	148
Total	48	32	200
Chi-square statistic = 0.71			
$p = 0.70$			
Tried Barbiturates			
Yes	4 (8%)	1 (3%)	
No	44	31	
Total	48	32	
Exact probability = 0.64			

[a] In the Rhode Island data, stimulants included "speed" and cocaine.

with increased drug or alcohol use in adolescence or young adult life.

We cannot emphasize enough that psychostimulant medications are not to be considered the sole method of treatment of attentional syndromes. When properly used as one of a spectrum of approaches, psychostimulant medication can help a child achieve success in school and acceptance by family and peers. With maturation, the need for medication appears to decrease, but some adolescents and young adults appear both to need the drugs and to derive continued benefit from its use.[14]

Although motor hyperactivity diminishes with age, a cognitive energy deficit and an inability or unwillingness to sustain attention may persist, which may be responsive to medication.

Weiss and associates[3] reported that 12 of 24 patients in early adolescence showed evidence of continued medication need when methylphenidate was withdrawn for study purposes, and Ackerman Dykman, and Peters[15] reported that 3 of 16 hyperactives were still on psychostimulants at the age of 14. We found that 10% of our mid-adolescent group needed psychostimulants to maintain acceptable academic performance. It is important to realize that the need for medication does not automatically disappear with puberty, and may continue into adult life.[14]

Adjustment in Adolescence

In their study, Ackerman, Dykman, and Peters[15] found that only 2 of 23 hyperactive adolescents presented no problem in the home, school, or community, and that nearly half presented fairly serious adjustment problems at age 14. We found that 46 of 81 youths (57%) presented no problems. Our results are similar to those reported by Mendelsohn, Johnson, and Stewart,[16] who found that half of the adolescents previously diagnosed as hyperactive were markedly improved. We found less antisocial behavior in our patients than did either Ackerman et al. or Mendelsohn and co-workers. It is most disturbing, however, to report the deaths of two adolescents in the immediate post-study period.

Young Adults

Our young adult studies are similar to the reports of Hechtman and associates[2] and of Borland and Heckman.[17]

Hechtman et al. reported that 35 subjects between the ages of 17 and 24 years, who had been diagnosed as hyperactive 10 years before, did not show significantly more antisocial behavior, non-medical use of drugs, or serious psychiatric disturbances than did a control group, although their tests of cognitive style indicated continued difficulty. Restlessness remained a problem, but their adjustment in work situations and living arrangements as comparable to that in the control population.

Borland and Heckman[17] showed that men who were hyperactive as boys 20–25 years previously did not experience serious social or psychiatric problems as adults. However, half of the group had minor psychiatric problems and they never achieved a socioeconomic status equal to that of their brothers.

Our young adults who had MBD had no major problems with adjustment, and their self-concept was normal, although lower than that of their siblings. Similarly, they had achieved a surprisingly high degree of education in view of their initial referral for school problems; it was, however, a lower level than their siblings achieved. Some continued to demonstrate impairment in short-term auditory memory (43%), visual perceptual problems (12.5%) and diadochokinetic skills (14%).

The impairments demonstrated are similar to those reported in learning disabled adolescents who may show choreiform movements, awkward skipping, dysdiadochokinesia, difficulties in imitation of finger movements, right-left confusion, and problems with the storage and retrieval of information, especially of a sequential nature.[15] However, these impairments rarely had the adverse effects in the adult world that they had had earlier in school situations.

When the Center was established, our goal was to assess each child's unique strengths and weaknesses and to devise therapeutic strategies designed to help him and his family cope with his individual school and personality problems. To achieve these objectives, the staff members were positive, nonjudgmental, optimistic, and patient advocates who helped parents fight for appropriate services in the community. Our aim was to change the perceptions about the child from "lazy" or "spoiled" to "frustrated," thus helping parents to gain a better appreciation of the difficulties their child faced in coping with an often arbitrary and overdemanding academic world.

When we could prevent the secondary emotional problems from developing in patients and their families, and do something positive in terms of mediation, time usually was an ally. When the reasons for failure could be traced, they often indicated a lack of or ineffective community support systems in education and mental health, and/or intractable family pathology.

Summary

One hundred and twenty-nine children diagnosed as having attentional disorders and related syndromes (minimal brain dysfunction and/or hyperkinetic behavior disorder) were studied during adolescence or young adulthood. Most had been treated with multiple therapeutic approaches which included psychostimulant medications. Forty-six of 81 adolescents (57%) were now problem-free. Thirteen (16 percent) of the remaining 35 youths were recommended for psychotherapy and 7 (8 percent) still required psychostimulant medication. Seven (8%) had developed significant antisocial problems and 2 (2%) others died of self-inflicted injuries. Forty-four (91 percent) of the 48 young adults were classified as successful, with normal self-concepts. They held jobs or were obtaining higher education. Twenty-one (43%) had poor short-term memory problems and 7 others (14%) considered themselves clumsy. There was no evidence to suggest that earlier chronic use of psychostimulant medication contributed to drug abuse. The incidence of alcoholism did not differ from that found in a normal control population.

Failures were in part related to both poor community support systems and/or intractable family pathology.

Appendix

Gross and Wilson Scale

0 Indicates no psychiatric impairment of any significance.
1 Refers to patients with such mild psychiatric impairment that some observers (family and/or teachers) would see a problem, while others would not.
2 Refers to patients in whom significant psychiatric impairment is demonstrated, but it is not incapacitating at all, although some definite disability is observable.
3 Refers to average psychiatric impairment, a fair degree of disability handicapping the child in his activities in a clear, perceptible way. Such a child would be considered by observers to have an impairment but would not be considered, for example, as the worst child in the class or the worst child on the block. This degree of impairment would be tolerable, if necessary, by both family and school.
4 Refers to more severe impairment, which is not tolerable by family or school. There would be considerable pressure on or by the family to do something about such a child.
5 Refers to a child who is barely supportable in the community. Such a child might be recommended for removal from the community but nevertheless be able to squeeze by. However, he is pinpointed by all concerned as a severe problem.
6 Refers to a child who is insupportable in the community and whose impairment is so great that hospitalization or institutionalization is necessary.

References

1. Menkes, M.M., Rowe, J.S., and Menkes, J.H.: A 25 year follow-up study on the hyperkinetic child with minimal brain dysfunction. *Pediatrics* **39:** 393, 1967.
2. Hechtman, L., Weiss, G., Finklestein, J., Werner, A., and Benn, R.: Hyperactives as young adults: A preliminary report. *Can Med Assoc J* **115:** 625, 1976.
3. Weiss, G., Kruger, E., Danielson, V., and Elman, M.: Effect of long-term treatment of hyperactive children with methylphenidate. *Can Med Assoc J* **112:** 159, 1975.
4. Laufer, M.W.: Long-term management and some follow-up findings on the use of drugs with minimal cerebral syndromes. *J Learn Disabil* **4:** 518, 1971.
5. Laufer, M.W., and Denhoff, E.: Hyperkinetic behavior syndrome in children. *J Pediatr* **50:** 463, 1959.
6. Clements, S.D.: Task force one: minimal brain dysfunction in children. National Institute of Neurological Diseases and Blindness, Monograph No. 3, U.S. Department of Health, Education and Welfare, Washington, D.C., 1966.
7. Werry, J.S.: Developmental hyperactivity. *Pediatr Clin North Am,* **15:** 581, 1968.
8. Gross, M., and Wilson, W.: *Minimal Brain Dysfunction.* Brunner Mazel, New York, 1974, pp. 15–16.
9. Fitts, W.H.: *Tennessee Self-Concept Scale Manual.* Nashville Counselor Recordings and Tests, Nashville, Tennessee, 1965.

10. *Drug Use in Rhode Island.* Health Planning Project, Community Medicine, Brown University, Providence, Rhode Island, March-April, 1976.
11. Slosson, R.L.: *Slosson Drawing Coordination Test (SDCT) for Children and Adults.* Slosson Educational Publications, East Aurora, New York.
12. Denhoff, E.: Locating young children with learning problems. *NY State J Med* **76:** 2007, 1976.
13. *Alcohol Use and Abuse under Age 25.* Community Medicine, Brown University, Providence Rhode Island, 1976.
14. Wood, D., Reimherr, F., Wender, P., and Johnson, G.: Diagnosis and treatment of minimal brain dysfunction in adults. *Arch Gen Psychiatry* **33:** 1453, 1976.
15. Ackerman, P., Dykman, R., and Peters, J.: Teenage status of hyperactive and non-hyperactive learning-disabled boys. *Am J Orthopsychiatry* **47:** 577, 1977.
16. Mendelsohn, W., Johnson, N., and Stewart, M.: Hyperactive children and teenagers: A follow-up study, *J Nerv Ment Dis* **153:** 273, 1971.
17. Borland, B., and Heckman, H.: Hyperactive boys and their brothers: A 25 year follow-up study. *Arch Gen Psychiatry* **33:** 669, 1976.

12

Cultural Variations in Perception and Management of Hyperactive Behavior

Lucile F. Newman, Ph.D.

The perception of hyperactivity is contingent on the complexity of society, and varies with an expansive world orientation and the values of individualism. Thus the term *hyperactive* becomes a cultural artifact, its definition emerging from a particular social situation, i.e., school, where the child's behavior is stressful to others, or other socially organized settings in which he is unable to control his own behavior to conform with social expectations. The term *dysfunction* suggests that we know more than we do about function: handedness, dominance, neural pathways. Whatever minimal brain dysfunction and hyperactivity are, they mean that something is not working right, and that it is not working socially.

One of the costs of social complexity is that we tolerate less and less in the way of individual variation. In an agrarian society children work outdoors, care for animals, and do regular chores. Education is only for those who want it or seem fit for it—by no means everyone. Given compulsory universal education, we tend to take children with widely varying visual and hearing perception, language capability, attention span, tolerance for immobility, and

---

Section on Community Health, Brown University, Providence, Rhode Island.

modes of learning and make them look as if they were all alike—sitting still, not talking or making trouble, focusing on a distant person or blackboard, and "learning."

What have other societies done about hyperactive behavior, or more likely, about children that were and are unusual? The literature of minimal brain dysfunction is for an anthropologist engaged in research or early human interaction, not one characterized by internal coherence. What we find is a common label for many slightly deviant functions—a catchall to enable the perception, categorizing, and management of uncontrollable behavior. And it is to break the downward spiral of behavior and response that therapeutic measures are taken. We do find common threads, however. One is the child's low self-esteem. Another is his experience, at least in time, of being at odds with the prevailing social expectations. Symptomatic behavior, as we might expect, varies. What appears to be the definitive concern of parents, teachers, and doctors is not that a child is overactive, but that he is uncontrollable by himself and others. It seems appropriate to discuss perception and management in this context as (1) cultural variation in perception of hyperactivity, and (2) cultural variation in management of socially difficult behavior.

Cultural Variation in Perception of Hyperactivity

Far from postulating any halcyon days when "noble savages" did better at things than we do now, it is necessary to point out that people who do not "fit in" to a particular society have always been a problem, and that ways of dealing with them have often been far from humane. The anthropological record, thin in this respect, is strongest in the collection and presentation of life history data, and the examples chosen will be from this literature. If we are discussing the treatment of children who provide problems to society, the human meaning of that treatment is never so clear as when it is expressed in their own words.

In some societies individualism is greatly valued and learning is perceived as focused on self-reliance and self-knowledge. The vision quest of American Indians of the Great Plains provides an example. It was an elaboration of solitary experience in which a child or adolescent left the social group in search of his or her own particular "vision." The experience was heightened by lack of food and sleep for perhaps days at a time, and was characterized by a seeking for a special experience, vision, or communication about what his or her future life was to be. It could sometimes occur during illness. Black Elk, an Oglala Sioux, described his vision experienced during a grave illness many years earlier in his childhood.

> Everybody was glad that I was living; but as I lay there thinking about the wonderful place where I had been and all that I had seen, I was very sad; for it seemed to me that everybody ought to know about it, but I was afraid to tell, because I knew that nobody would believe me, little as I was, for I was only nine years old. Also, as I lay there thinking of my vision, I could see it all again and feel the meaning with a part of me like a strange power glowing in my body; but when the part of me that talks would try to make words for the meaning, it would be like fog and get away from me.
>
> I am sure now that I was then too young to understand it all, and that I only felt it. It was the pictures I remembered and the words that went with them; for nothing I have ever seen with my eyes was so clear and bright as what my vision showed me; and no words that I have ever heard with my ears were like the words I heard. I did not have to remember these things; they have remembered themselves all these years.[2]

This was the single dominating educational experience of his life. It accomplished identity formation, establishment of future occupation, and the acquisition of a personal community of animal spirits sacred to him alone. It was an individualized environment for learning structured by the cultural expectations, and attuned to the abilities, needs, and understanding of the individual. The vision quest is not institutionalized as it used to be, but it still figures in the dreams and play of American Indian children. This is mentioned because among native Americans forced into the prevailing "Anglo" school system, there is a high incidence in the schoolroom of what is defined as MBD syndrome.

Cultural Variation in Management of Socially Difficult Behavior

Forms of social control vary by cultural heritage and differ greatly according to prevailing values and definitions of what is perceived as normal for a particular society. Many forms of social control are stringent, painful, and damaging. Some of them may be described in terms of isolation or of labeling.

Isolation

Isolation and sometimes ostracism may be accomplished within the family, as has been described in the traditional Chinese family.

"Through the system of mutual responsibility (the so-called *pao chia* system) individuals were responsible for each others' actions within the household, and families were responsible for one another within a community, much as in Communist China today. It is a story of family system hierarchies and authoritarianism."[3] To quote Maxine Hong Kingston, in *The Woman Warrior* ". . . when my mother and father talked about their life back home sometimes they mentioned an 'outcast table'. . . . In a commensal tradition where food is precious, the powerful older people made wrongdoers eat alone. Instead of letting them start separate new lives like the Japanese, who could become samurais or geishas, the Chinese family, faces averted but eyes glowering sideways, hung onto the offenders and fed them leftovers." And again, Reischauer and Fairbank: ". . . an insubordinate child might be severely punished. In times of stress, parents might even sell or give away their intractable children."[3] Social control was accomplished at home. Behavior of any member reflected on the family and was modified there. Manners, including those of deference and demeanor, were extremely important. A severely deviant child might never be seen outside the family, but might also be isolated within it.

Labeling

In many societies the child whose rhythms are out of synchrony with those around him may be labeled a "spirit child," a witch, a person potentially to be feared. As in all labeling, the name permits authoritative action in terms of the label and the child may suffer extreme punishment or ostracism as a result of it. In the religious model, a child may be perceived as being possessed of the devil or demons and may be subjected to exorcism.

We, similarly, manage some kinds of difficult or uncontrollable behavior by labeling the child as *sick* and the control of this behavior as *therapy*, thereby leaving the educational institutions intact and, in many cases, abrogating the responsibility to actually teach children. Should we perhaps question the existing institutions rather than modify the children to fit them?

What, then, can these comparisons suggest to us? First, they can suggest that nonconforming and uncontrollable behaviors are particularly problematic in a complex society and less so in agrarian societies or those less characterized by concentrations of population. Second, it has been suggested before, but should be reiterated, that we are all too ready to modify the child or his behavior. It is time to reexamine the institutions in which he finds himself. Have we, for example, considered following the example of some Eastern European countries and beginning school at 8 years of age, thereby preventing the problem of forcing immature bodies and minds into adult modes of attention? Finally, now that we are beginning to understand something of modes of learning and the immense individual variations in cognitive functioning and how children learn, would it not be possible to consider translating that understanding into new institutional forms for teaching and learning?

References

1. Kingston, M.H.: *The Woman Warrior*. Alfred Knopf, New York, 1976, p. 7.
2. Neihardt, J.G.: *Black Elk Speaks*. Pocket Books, New York, 1972, pp. 40–41.
3. Reischauer, E.O., and Fairbank, J.K.: *East Asia: The Great Tradition*. Houghton Mifflin, Boston, 1960, pp. 28, 29.
4. Benedict, R.: The vision quest. In *An Anthropologist at Work*, M. Mead, Ed. Houghton Mifflin, Boston, 1959, p. 18.

13

Behavior Disorders and Learning Disabilities in a Rural Environment Treatment and Long-Term Outcome

Hans R. Huessy, M.D.

This chapter reports our experiences with minimal brain dysfunction over the years in rural Vermont, an area where the problem is not complicated by problems of race, major poverty, or ghettos. We began our studies by surveying all the elementary school children in the first six grades in one county, asking the teachers to identify all the children they were concerned about. The results are seen in Figure 1. The four major complaints accounted for 80 percent of all the children that the schools were concerned about. This was rather surprising to us, since we had not thought that minimal brain dysfunction was the predominant difficulty among elementary school children. The teachers were concerned about 20% of all the children.

We then did an 8- to 10-year follow-up study of 84 children, seen by us in the past, whom we thought suitable for drug therapy. The outcomes were not very promising. Of the 84 children, 9 could not be located, 18 had been institutionalized, and 5 had been in two or more institutions. The school dropout rate was 21 percent, versus the expected rate of 4 percent. Twenty-four had satisfactory and 13 had poor work records. There was no relationship between drug response

---

Professor of Psychiatry, University of Vermont; Outpatient Psychiatry Service, DeGoesbriand Unit, Medical Center Hospital of Vermont, Burlington, Vermont.

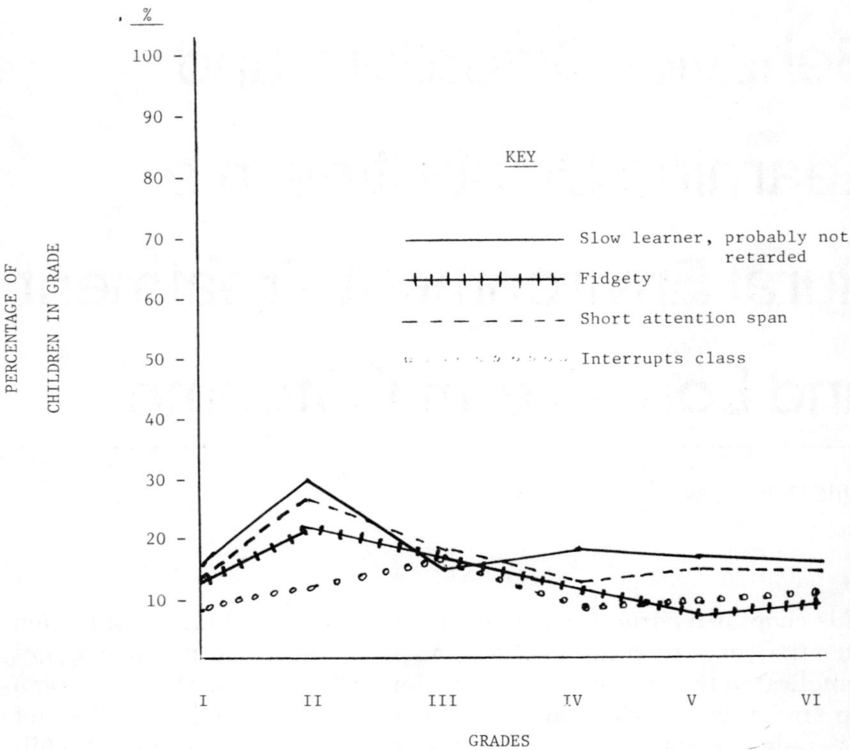

Figure 1. Major problems displayed by 1113 schoolchildren (grades 1–6) in Addison County, Vermont.

or length of use and outcome. We interpreted these data as indicating that the child with MBD is indeed a child at risk for all kinds of later disorders.

In our next study teachers filled out a questionnaire concerning 500 second-grade children in a number of rural schools. This questionnaire was then completed by the children's fourth and fifth grade teachers, after which we examined the children's adjustment in the ninth grade. These questionnaires rated children in regard to hyperkinetic behavior and learning problems. The greater the problems, the higher the score. By rather arbitrary means we decided that all the children with scores above the 80th percentile showed behavior usually identified with the MBD syndrome. The results of this study are presented in Table 1. Children identified in second, fourth, and fifth

TABLE 1
Results of the Study

Group	Above 80th Percentile	No. of Children	Boys Percent	Mean IQ Scores	Grade Point Average	Percent of Group in Remedial Math	Percent of Group in Remedial English	Percent of Group in Advanced Math	Percent of Group in Advanced English	Percent of Children who Repeated One or More Grades	Percent of Children with Poor or Very Poor Social Adjustment
A	2nd grade only	17	60	97.8	2.22	47	24	6	6	47	0
B	4th grade only	14	57	97.3	1.89	25	16	17	0	43	23
C	5th grade only	17	76	98.4	1.93	31	50	0	0	29	59
D	2nd and 4th grades	13	62	90.0	1.95	45	18	0	0	82	25
E	2nd and 5th grades	10	70	83.9	1.90	44	55	0	0	67	20
F	4th and 5th grades	14	93	96.9	1.68	33	75	0	0	62	54
G	2nd, 4th and grades	10	100	90.0	1.48	44	67	0	0	33	70
All Identified Children		95	73	95.3	1.90	38	42	5	1	50	35
All Controls		45	67	107.3	2.76	2	14	27	23	11	7
	Percentile										
H	0–30	22	68	114.1	2.97	0	5	36	32	0	0
I	40–70	23	65	100.7	2.55	5	23	18	14	22	13

grade as showing symptoms of MBD had serious problems in ninth grade. Children who were identified as having MBD only in the second grade were doing quite well, although not nearly as well as children who showed no symptoms of MBD. Children who received consistently low scores, i.e., in the lower 30 percentiles on all three teacher questionnaires, had an unusually high level of adaptation with no social or academic problems, at least one-third of them being in advanced classes in either English or math. The study seems to show that children who show MBD behavior for more than 1 year, particularly at the fourth and fifth grade level, are a population at risk for later difficulties. We used MBD as a label without any commitment to a specific causality or therapy.

Table 2 shows some clusters that we obtained from the data. A score of 66 was at the 80th percentile. As can be seen, we were able to find five groups that seemed to have stability over time, with the first cluster becoming progressively worse, the third cluster showing gradual improvement, and the other three clusters showing stability over time. We would like to be able to differentiate the high-scoring second-grader who will improve from the one who will get worse, but so far we cannot.

We then looked at these children's school records in the twelfth grade. Again, the children who had had scores above the 80th percentile had poorer adjustments in every area than children who never scored above the 80th percentile (see Table 3).

After we began this research, Conners developed his by now standard questionnaire for both parents and teachers, which has been found to be the most useful diagnostic tool for MBD. To see how well our questionnaire correlated with the one developed by Dr. Conners, the teachers of 350 third- and fourth-graders filled out both question-

TABLE 2
Analysis of Total Scores with Five Clusters

Cluster Number	*Number of Subjects*		*2nd Grade*	*Cluster Centers 4th Grade*	*5th Grade*
1	36		65.0	69.6	76.5
2	57		54.9	57.3	60.9
3	38		69.9	62.3	55.9
4	60		49.8	49.5	47.8
5	51		39.5	37.7	36.6
		Mean	54.3	53.8	54.1
		SD	12.0	12.6	14.0

For all practical purposes a score of 66 represents the 80th percentile in each case.

TABLE 3
Results in the Twelfth Grade

	Percent with poor Social Adjustment	*Percent in Remedial*		*Percent in Advanced*		*Mean Grade*		
		English	*Math*	*English*	*Math*	*English*	*Math*	*GPA*
No scores in 80th percentile	12	6	5	25	35	2.67	2.64	2.73
One or more scores in 80th percentile	29	11	12	2	0	1.76	1.54	1.79

naires. We found that we achieved a correlation coefficient of 0.77 and that our questionnaire selected some children with educational handicaps who were not picked up by the Conners questionnaire. Conners himself states that he feels his questionnaire is deficient in singling out children with educational handicaps.

Table 4 summarizes the ways in which the hyperkinetic children were described in their ninth grade records and contains only items which are not found at all in the ninth grade records of children who never achieved a score above the 80th percentile. There appear to be three predictive factors: fidgetiness, a "nuisance" factor, and a factor related to poor learning. The combination of all three factors is a far superior predictor of later performance than any one alone. The descriptions make clear that these children are different. We tried various different percentiles as cutoff points for segregating the problem children from the nonproblem children; as originally noted, however, the 80th percentile remained the best cutoff point.

A further finding is that, rather than there being MBD children and non-MBD children, the behaviors picked up by these questionnaires are distributed on a standard curve of distribution (see Fig. 2). Our clinical experience clearly shows that children can move up and down this curve in response to various environmental factors. In

TABLE 4
Descriptions of Hyperkinetic Children in the Ninth Grade Who Were Suspended, Placed on Social Probation, or Assigned Detention

Offenses committed:	Teachers considered them:
Truancy	Loud
Tardiness	Inattentive
Smoking in school	Uncooperative
Cutting classes	Lazy
Forging passes	Sneaky
Stealing	Immature
Discharging fire extinguishers	Annoying
Disrupting the classroom	Inconsiderate
Defying school authorities	Unpredictable
	Defiant
	Easily discouraged
	Easily distracted
	In addition, teachers noted:
	Daydreaming
	Fooling around
	Disturbing others
	Seeking attention
	Responding poorly to discipline
	Inability to sit still, concentrate, settle down, and/or follow directions

None of the records of the control population contained comments similar to these.

our attempts to treat these children, we found that they often responded to small doses of imipramine, and we reported this in 1970.[2]

The results of these studies led us to look for adult hyperkinetics. Table 5 shows the results of 142 drug trials in 64 adults who had symptoms or childhood histories of MBD. The results show that adults with these symptoms respond very much as children do, and also that the variability of response is similar to that in children, namely children may respond to one of the stimulant drugs but not to another and there is no way of predicting which medication a particular individual will respond to.

As part of this study, we came upon the interesting finding that women with MBD seem to be particularly sensitive to fluid retention before their menstrual periods and may receive dramatic help from the use of a diuretic. We found that stimulants were seldom needed in such patients.

The fear that these drugs interfere with height and weight gains is not borne out by our own data. These children are characterized by erratic height and weight curves, making this question an extremely difficult one to answer with any certainty.

The opinion that only early aggressive behavior indicates a poor prognosis is widely held. The studies above would not bear this out. Table 6 summarizes some of the environmental factors which our experience has shown either aggravate or improve the behavior of children with MBD. It helps to explain why MBD presents a much greater problem in the United States than in Western Europe and, in turn, a greater problem in Western Europe than in more rigidly organized societies. The diversity in our society, the various acceptable life-styles, and our tendency toward the open classroom all make life more difficult for the child with MBD. It would appear that the problem is becoming greater in Western Europe as the social structure becomes more varied.

Table 7 lists the different presenting behaviors at different ages for MBD. The work of several investigators[7,8–9,10] makes it clear that we could identify many of these children very early in life. The question is What should we be doing about it? Does early treatment alter adult outcome? Is there a time after which treatment is pointless? If it is symptom control only, does prolonged control of symptoms alter final outcome? Our experience with adults leads us to postulate that a crucial dimension in MBD has to do with the individual's relationship to time. These children and adults live in the present. We have experienced adults, whose behavior was greatly improved by medication, coming back and saying that they would not take the medication anymore. Whereas the drug abuser uses medication to

TABLE 5
Results of 142 Drug Trials in 64 Adults with Symptoms or a History of MBD

	Imipramine (Tofranil)	*Amiptryptyline (Elavil)*	*Methylphenidate (Ritalin)*	*Dextroamphetamine (Dexedrine)*	*Diphenylhydantoin (Dilantin)*	*Pemoline (Cylert)*	*Methamphetamine (Desoxyn)*	*Total*
No. of trials	55	26	28	17	13	2	1	142
No. of positive responses	26	12	13	9	7	0	1	68
No. of negative responses	10	7	6	3	2	1	0	29
No. of paradoxical negative responses	1	0	1	0	1	0	0	3
No. of no effect responses	21	8	9	5	5	1	0	49
No. of responses with positive-negative aspects	3	1	1	0	2	0	0	7
Percent positive responses	47.3	46.2	46.4	52.9	53.8	0	100	47.9
Dosage for Males — Range (mg)	50–150	50–125	30–100	10–30	200–400	—	—	
Dosage for Males — Mean (mg)	90.9	90.6	56.7	16.2	300	—	—	
Dosage for Females — Range (mg)	25–150	50–125	15–100	10–30	100–300	—	10	
Dosage for Females — Mean (mg)	74.0	78.1	42.5	20.0	200	—	10	

TABLE 6
Environmental Factors that Affect MBD

Factors that Aggravate MBD	*Factors that Improve MBD*
Large family	Small family
No extended family	Extended family available
Frequent moves	Much large muscle activity
Apartment living	Rigid social structure
Trailer living	Fully scheduled day
Emphasis on formal education	Single family home
Open and diverse society	One-to-one teaching
Frequent conflicting messages	Tightly run classroom
Much free time	
Open classroom	

TABLE 7
Behaviors Associated with MBD at Various Stages of Life

Infancy	*Preschool*	*Elementary School*
Restlessness	*Into everything*	*Short attention span*
Irritability	Short attention span	Daydreams (girls)
Irregularity	*Destructive*	Can't sit still (boys)
Excessive crying	Can't sit still	Low frustration tolerance
High fevers	Temper tantrums	*Overreacts*
Poor eater	Speech problems	*Learning problems*
High activity level	Gets to sleep or wakes up very early	Doesn't complete tasks
	Cruelty to animals	Class clown
	Aggressive	Aggressive
	Impulsive	Poor peer relations
	Trouble with groups	Impulsive
	Mood swings	Poor self-image
	Fire setting	
	Enuresis	

High School	*Adulthood*
Educationally retarded	Easily distractible
Poor attention span	Impulsive
Lack of motivation	*Short fuse*
Unreliable	Explosive
Aggressive	Sleep problems
Impulsive	Mood swings
Overreacts	*Trouble with lasting relationships*
Struggles with authority	*Can't relax*
Delinquent activity (boys)	Stretches the truth
Promiscuity (girls)	Trouble with groups
Mood swings	Alcohol abuse
Lies	Overly dramatic
Accident prone	*Poor self-image*
Suicidal gestures	Exposes self
Poor self-image	Poor job performance
School drop out	Frequent arguments or fights

"tune out" temporarily and to live for the moment, the MBD person, if the medication works, is prevented from living in the moment. Apparently, if one has not grown up with an internal tolerance for stress and frustration, when medication suddenly gives one this privilege, it is not particularly attractive. Our patients never want more. They continually want to stop taking medication. None of them appear to want to become responsible. One question we cannot answer at all yet is whether age influences which drug may help.

Since a tight social structure helps these individuals get along better, our negative attitude toward institutions may reflect our prejudices more than reality. A tightly run institution may be the best treatment for one of these children. The institution should not be a place to hold the child so that treatment can be applied; rather, the institution itself should be the treatment.

Table 8 shows the standard curve of distribution of MBD behaviors and shows factors which have been shown to be associated with the prevalence of MBD. The fact that MBD has a better outcome in families of higher socioeconomic status is related to the resources available to help parents deal with a difficult situation. The same is true in cases of perinatal insult.

The usual model is a problem family producing a problem child. We would say that often a problem child may produce a problem family. Although we do not have the evidence, we believe that allowing one of these children to go through school with reasonable academic and social success should produce a better outcome than having the child continually in academic and social difficulty. For this reason we are very ready to use medication if it helps.

Among the adult outcomes of this disorder are alcoholism, criminality, and hysterical personality, conditions for which we have few treatment resources. Many of these individuals show serious deficiencies in their ability to form lasting relationship, which may be one of the most important prognostic indicators. Is this disability based on the symptoms of MBD, i.e., is it the result of MBD, or is it an essential ingredient of MBD or only some cases of MBD? If MBD is largely hereditary, than this would account for the higher incidence of maladaptive problems among adopted children. Adolescents with MBD are more likely to become involved in illegitimate pregnancy. Since most adopted children are the result of illegitimate pregnancies, they therefore would have an unusually heavy genetic loading for MBD. Individuals with MBD do not achieve as high a socioeconomic status as their non-MBD siblings. They drop out of school, get involved at a high rate in delinquency and crime, and have unstable job histories, so they will be overrepresented among the poor.

TABLE 8

←	→
Stable environment	Complications of pregnancy and delivery
Adequate economic resources	Poverty
Well established routines	Prematurity
Predictable and consistent consequences	Instability of parents
Parental stability	Open, unstructured environment
Well structured school system	Inconsistent discipline
	Environmental disruption
	Injuries and infections of brain

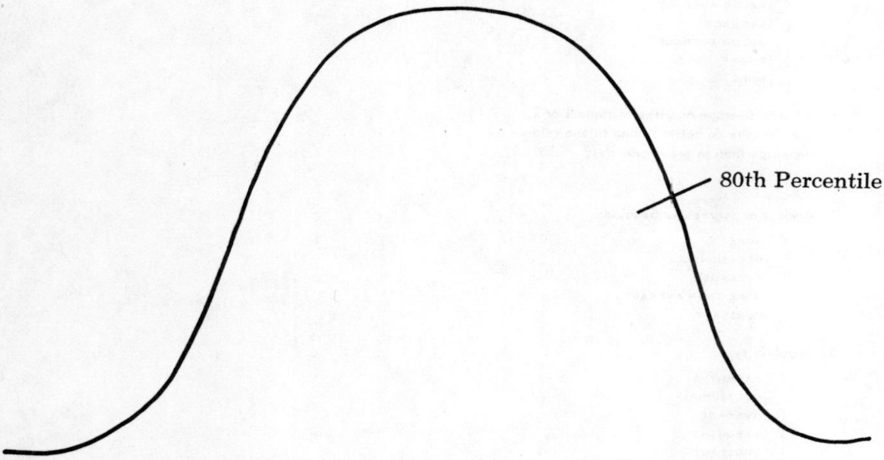

Further, poor prenatal, perinatal, and postnatal care is much more common among the poor and, again, is strongly associated with MBD. Prematurity is more common among the poor and is also associated with MBD. (Smoking and drinking in mothers have been shown to have negative influences on their offspring. Excesses in both of these activities are more likely in MBD than in normal adults.) Therefore, we know of many factors which contribute to the overrepresentation of the MBD syndrome among the poor. MBD as described in this paper accounts for 80% of the school-age problem children. It represents a population at risk for various negative adult outcomes which cost society a great deal in all ways. We can now identify the person with MBD quite early in life; the challenge is to show that we can do something for these children and alter their dismal futures.

Appendix

HUESSY PSYCHIATRIC HISTORY

Name: ____________________ Birthday: ____________

Sex: ____________

I. SOCIAL MATURITY: *REMARKS*

1. Degree of participation in group activities.
   - [ ] ABOVE AVERAGE
   - [ ] AVERAGE
   - [ ] BELOW AVERAGE
   - [ ] POOR
   - [ ] NONE

2. Relationship to adults and children on a one to one basis.
   - [ ] ABOVE AVERAGE
   - [ ] AVERAGE
   - [ ] BELOW AVERAGE
   - [ ] POOR
   - [ ] NONE

3. If below average on either ratings 1 or 2, does he/she do better in one to one relationships than in group settings?
   - [ ] YES [ ] NO

4. Amount of aggressive behavior.
   - [ ] NONE
   - [ ] OCCASIONAL
   - [ ] AVERAGE
   - [ ] MORE THAN AVERAGE
   - [ ] CONSTANT

5. Impulsivity.
   - [ ] RARELY
   - [ ] OCCASIONAL
   - [ ] AVERAGE
   - [ ] FREQUENT
   - [ ] CONSTANT

6. Frustration tolerance.
   - [ ] UNUSUALLY HIGH TOLERANCE
   - [ ] FAIRLY HIGH TOLERANCE
   - [ ] AVERAGE TOLERANCE
   - [ ] MODERATELY LOW TOLERANCE
   - [ ] VERY LOW TOLERANCE

7. Overall emotional mood.
   - [ ] FLUCTUATES APPROPRIATE TO SURROUNDINGS AND SUBJECT MATERIAL WITH KEEN INTEREST
   - [ ] FLUCTUATES APPROPRIATELY, BUT LESS INTENSELY THAN ABOVE
   - [ ] FLUCTUATES ACCORDING TO INTEREST AND STIMULI
   - [ ] REQUIRES ADDITIONAL STIMULUS TO GET DESIRED RESPONSE
   - [ ] SEVERE FLUCTUATIONS IN MOOD, FROM ECSTASY TO DEEP DESPAIR WITH LITTLE STIMULUS

8. Parents and other teachers report problems with this child with frequent crisis situations occurring.
   - [ ] NEVER
   - [ ] RARELY
   - [ ] FREQUENTLY
   - [ ] QUITE FREQUENTLY
   - [ ] CONSTANTLY

Page 2

REMARKS

II. NERVOUS AND MUSCULAR DEVELOPMENT:

1. Coordination and agility.
   - ☐ SUPERIOR
   - ☐ GOOD
   - ☐ AVERAGE
   - ☐ POOR
   - ☐ VERY POOR

2. Fine muscle tremor and/or twitches of face, hands and arms are noted (i.e. fidgity).
   - ☐ NEVER
   - ☐ RARELY
   - ☐ OCCASIONALLY
   - ☐ FREQUENTLY
   - ☐ CONSTANTLY

3. Speech and ability to express himself are
   - ☐ SUPERIOR
   - ☐ ABOVE AVERAGE
   - ☐ AVERAGE
   - ☐ BELOW AVERAGE
   - ☐ POOR

4. Writing ability is
   - ☐ EXCELLENT
   - ☐ ABOVE AVERAGE
   - ☐ AVERAGE
   - ☐ POOR
   - ☐ UNREADABLE

III. PERFORMANCE:

1. Spatial perception and ability to see and correct errors.
   - ☐ SUPERIOR
   - ☐ ABOVE AVERAGE
   - ☐ AVERAGE
   - ☐ POOR
   - ☐ VERY POOR

2. Reading level according to age and grade.
   - ☐ SUPERIOR
   - ☐ ABOVE AVERAGE
   - ☐ AVERAGE
   - ☐ BELOW AVERAGE
   - ☐ VERY RETARDED

3. Mathematics level according to age and grade.
   - ☐ SUPERIOR
   - ☐ ABOVE AVERAGE
   - ☐ AVERAGE
   - ☐ BELOW AVERAGE
   - ☐ VERY RETARDED

4. Spelling level according to age and grade.
   - ☐ SUPERIOR
   - ☐ ABOVE AVERAGE
   - ☐ AVERAGE
   - ☐ BELOW AVERAGE
   - ☐ VERY RETARDED

5. Performance in general is
   - ☐ SUPERIOR
   - ☐ ABOVE AVERAGE
   - ☐ AVERAGE
   - ☐ CONSISTANTLY POOR
   - ☐ VERY UNPREDICTABLE AND ERRATIC

Page 3

REMARKS

IV. GENERAL ATTITUDE AND BEHAVIOR:

1. Activity and energy level seems
   - [ ] ABOVE AVERAGE AND WELL ORGANIZED
   - [ ] AVERAGE
   - [ ] ANNOYING AND FAIRLY POORLY ORGANIZED
   - [ ] LOW ENERGY AND POORLY ORGANIZED
   - [ ] CONSTANT MOTION AS THOUGH DRIVEN

2. Interest span
   - [ ] CONCENTRATES TO THE EXCLUSION OF OUTSIDE DISTRACTIONS
   - [ ] COMPLETES TASKS WELL
   - [ ] NEEDS URGING TO STICK WITH A TASK
   - [ ] IS EASILY DISTRACTED
   - [ ] JUMPS FROM ONE ACTIVITY TO ANOTHER WITHOUT COMPLETING ANY (SHORT INTEREST SPAN)

3. In permissive or group activities
   - [ ] REMAINS ORGANIZED AND LEADS
   - [ ] COOPERATIVE WITH OTHERS AND LEADERS
   - [ ] BEHAVIOR VARIES LITTLE FROM STRUCTURED SETTING
   - [ ] TENDS TO BE OVEREXCITED AND LOSE CONTROL
   - [ ] BECOMES EXCITED TO THE ECSTATIC POINT

4. Personality
   - [ ] LOVEABLE
   - [ ] LIKEABLE
   - [ ] NEUTRAL
   - [ ] OFTEN ANNOYING
   - [ ] UNPREDICTABLE

5. Intelligence (your judgement, not I.Q.)
   - [ ] SUPERIOR
   - [ ] ABOVE AVERAGE
   - [ ] AVERAGE
   - [ ] BELOW AVERAGE
   - [ ] VERY DULL

References

1. Huessy, H.R.: Study of the prevalence and therapy of the choreatiform syndrome or hyperkinesis in rural Vermont. *Acta Paedopsychiatr* **34:** 130–135, 1967.
2. Huessy, H.R., and Gendron, R.M.: Prevalence of the so-called hyperkinetic syndrome in public school children of Vermont. *Acta Paedopsychiatr* **37:** 243–248, 1970.
3. Huessy, H.R., Marshall, C.D., and Gendron, R.A.: Five hundred children followed from grade 2 through grade 5 for the prevalence of behavior disorder. *Acta Paedopsychiatr* **39:** 301–309, 1973.
4. Huessy, H.R., Metoyer, M., and Townsend, M.: 8–10 year follow-up of 84 children treated for behavioral disorder in rural Vermont. *Acta Paedopsychiatr* **40:** 230–235, 1974.

5. Huessy, H.R., and Cohen, A.H.: Hyperkinetic behaviors and learning disabilities followed over seven years. *Pediatrics* **57:** 4–10, 1976.
6. Huessy, H.R., and Blair, C.L.: Clinical trials of drug therapy in 64 adults with symptoms and/or childhood histories of minimal brain dysfunction. (Unpublished.)
7. Prechtl, H.F.R.: Neurological findings in newborn infants after pre- and perinatal complications. Groningen Nutricia Symposium, Aspects of Praematurity and Dysmaturity, May 1967.
8. Waldrop, M., and Halverson, C.: Minor physical anomalies and hyperactive behavior in young children. *In The Exceptional Infant*. Brunner/Mazel, New York, 1971, p. 34.
9. Thomas, R., Chess, S., and Birch, H.: *Temperament and Behavior Disorders in Children*. New York University Press, New York, 1968.
10. Brazelton, T.B.: Implications of infant development among the Mayan Indians of Mexico. *Hum Dev* **15:** 90–111, 1972.
11. Conners, C.K.: A teacher rating scale for use in drug studies with children. *Am J Psychiatry* **126:** 884–888, 1969.

14

The Educator Views Hyperactivity, Learning, and Medication

Harry S. Novack, Ph.D.

My business is helping school age children who do not, cannot, or will not meet the expectations of their environment and who as a result are labeled as learning disabled, hyperkinetic, having minimal brain dysfunction, etc. I have been teaching, testing, and researching these youngsters and their educational systems for some years. The approach to these children has been influenced by association with colleagues from a wide variety of disciplines—audiology and speech pathology, child psychiatry, child neurology—and, in recent years, by a rigorous statistician and research psychologist, and by a clinical educator of great ability. It is from this extensive interaction that I would like to address several of the subtopics concerning MBD and to consider with you factors which I believe have adversely affected most of the research dealing with learning disabilities and hyperkinesis.

For one thing, it appears that we are dealing with what is essentially a middle-class phenomenon. It is rare to find children other than from a middle-lass environment who have either the luxury or the misfortune of being diagnosed and labeled in these terms.

Professor of Special Education, Rhode Island College, Providence, Rhode Island.

Lower-class children sometimes get these labels when they are looked at in a clinic by middle-class physicians. How did this trend come about? One might say that the story of learning disabilities and hyperkinesis, at least from the point of view of the psychologist and educator, began when Alfred Strauss, influenced by the work of Kurt Goldstein, attempted to relate the behavior shown by some children to that of the brain-injured soldiers of World War I. There began over 40 years in which research aimed to prove that the incessant activity and/or inappropriate behavior of children was the result of damage, infection, or malfunctioning at various levels of the central nervous system. In the absence of specific evidence for such relationships, physicians began to scale down the abnormality of the central nervous system from brain damage to brain injury to brain dysfunction to other types suboptimal functioning as yet unnamed. Today many researchers are using poorly defined terms to designate various populations of children whose behavior is considered lacking or inappropriate. These investigators are trying to affect unilateral, one-to-one connections between causes and behavior where none currently appear to exist. In the meantime, during this 40-year period, by accident or by design, medication was introduced to treat this phenomenon of hyperactivity.

Five years ago, I pointed out that the results of the research with some medications were quite nebulous and inconsistent.[6] The problems, of course, were that the populations studied were small and vaguely described, the age range was too heterogenous, the methods of handling and reporting data were vague, and the results drawn were often inappropriate. It appeared that most of the research was being done by clinical physicians with the help of psychologists who had minimal knowledge or appreciation for the research process. Why do physicians always assume that all phychologists are researchers? Too often, psychologists permit physicians to ultize data obtained under the pressure to respond to the hopes, fears, and failures of both parents and educators shirking their duty. The decision to prescribe medication is rarely made on the basis of firsthand observation of behavior in the environment in which one does not function well, nor on the basis of solid medical evidence. The physician, according to his ability, interest, time and sophistication, makes his decision. The evidence seems to suggest that medication for behavior management is still a treatment to be used with clinical skill and expertise.

It would appear that most decisions about medication are derived from an insufficient research base and applied to populations which, thus far, have eluded precise definition. Take for example the so-called learning disabled child: As of December 1, 1976, the Department of Health, Education, and Welfare was still unable to define learning disabled children. In fact, after all these years, DHEW had asked for an additional 90 days, hoping to come up with a definition by April 1, 1977. In the *Federal Register* of that earlier date, the agency reported that among the factors delaying its ability to arrive at a conclusive definition was the fact that it had to deal with data supplied by one individual who had identified "99 different minimal brain dysfunctions."

In working with school children and their teachers, a true understanding of learning disability requires that we eliminate many of the conditions in our schools which adversely affect the learning potential of all children. Schools are not kind places to children who do not learn readily. Until recently, most schools were determined not to provide alternatives to such children. This is quite ominous when one considers the data of Katrina DeHirsch,[8] who found that 40–60% of all children entering the first grade were not ready to learn nor to profit from traditionally available materials and methods. It is only now, through legislative pressure and with more money being allotted for special education, that schools are attempting to resolve this problem. However, neither the schools nor the teachers have the appropriate know-how to effect this change. They have been poorly equipped for this purpose by our teacher training institutions, staffed for the most part by educators lacking any appreciation, patience, or understanding for children who can't learn easily. Many children are labeled learning disabled because of the narrow training of their teachers, who show great agility in calling for medication and fancy labels to explain pathology and failure to learn. Why does the problem usually appear when the child starts school? Why is it that so many children on medication do not need to use their medication during the summer vacations? Where and why did the hyperactivity or hyperkinesis suddenly go?

During the past 4 years, a colleague and I have examined the many studies on hyperkinesis. The controversy and the semantic confusion which the word generates reflects the chaotic state which exists in the literature. Hyperkinesis still has not been precisely defined, with as many points of view as there are researchers. Each, unfortunately, rarely considers the possibility that the problem of hyperkinesis is representative of factors that extend beyond the boundaries of one point of view. We have adopted a more flexible, or "electric," perspective of hyperkinesis, which holds that in addition to perceiving the problem of *exclusive* etiology, there is a need for an *inclusive* approach, one which neither negates nor restricts the current prevailing theories. While many might accept this premise academically or intellectually, few treatment or research aspects support this concept.

Most of the theories concerning etiology and subsequent behavioral correlates can be placed within three major groupings. There are those who maintain that hyperkinesis or hyperactivity is a constitutional phenomenon, that there is something in a child's physical make-up that predisposes him to this behavior. However, even under this explanatory umbrella of constitutional or physiologic causalities, the causes themselves are subjects of wide disagreement.[5]

A second group emphasizes that hyperactivity is a form of learned behavior. Its onset becomes established as a reaction to specific conditions which then becomes generalized to other situations. Within one school of learning theory, the opinion is forwarded that hyperactivity stems from the very naming or diagnosis of this phenomenon. More simply, the child's behavior is identified by someone within his environment—parent, teacher, or even physician—as hyperkinetic. The label is then affixed to the child, creating a continuing stigma under which the child is thereafter known and treated as hyperactive. The child, in turn, learns to behave just as he is perceived by those around him, thus enacting a kind of self-fulfilling prophecy.[2]

The third major group presents hyperkinesis as the manifestation of a personality disorder. Most psychiatrists and other professionals from the field of mental health, such as social workers and clinical psychologists, would view the issue from this perspective, agreeing that hyperkinesis is a reflection of a child's inner conflict and anxiety and that it is primarily emotionally based.[1]

Within the areas of research and treatment, these theories of etiology are considered mutually exclusive. In contrast, an eclectic orientation holds that hyperkinesis is rarely caused by physiologic or psychoemotional factors existing in isolation. The physical child is viewed as interacting with his envioronment and, more often than not, it is a combination of both his nature and his nurture which may precipitate and perpetuate the behavior known as hyperkinesis.

This eclectic point of view fits easily within the theoretical framework of Kurt Lewin's field theory.[4] He suggests that behavior is a function of a person's interaction with his environment. When applied to hyperkinesis, one might then state that the behavior known as hyperactivity may be a manifestation of the physical component of the child, interacting with his total environment.

Further, we see hyperkinesis as emerging in part or wholly from *certain interplays* of environmental situations and physical states. These situations include: (1) A developmental period when some children may have trouble becoming organized or attentive to some selective stimuli. (2) During this same period children are subject to a variety of stressful forces; for example, competition from siblings, demands and expectations from parents, situations in which they receive too little or inadequate attention, times when their behavior or speech is unnecessarily and frequently interrupted, and unstable environments which may be lacking in consistent or reasonable expectations. Schools do a good job here—making some children work at their frustration level. (3) Particularly vulnerable children have a low frustration tolerance and are less hardy than other children in assimilating or integrating physiologic or psychological stress. (4) There are various subcultures, in our case the broad middle-class, which emphasize rules of social deportment at too early an age for some children. This last point may account for the discrepancies observed in this country as compared with the Isle of Wight, where, in a study of over 2200 children between the ages of 5 and 15, only five hyperkinetics were found.[7]

Many children may experience one or even two of these situations without suffering any ill effects. It is their occurrence in combination at significant times which may spawn the syndrome labeled hyperkinesis. To refer back to Lewin's formula, $B = f(p \times e)$, we suggest that within broad limits, hyperactivity may be elicited or diminished by affecting the physical dimension of the person or the psychological and social environment in which he finds himself.

We have found this paradigm valid for other conditions of behavior. It has been observed in dealing with mental retardation that often we can change some of the dimensions of the retardation. For example, it has been shown that removing children from institutions or keeping them out of institutions, results in IQs higher than those of children who have been institutionalized. There is also evidence that retarded children reared in foster homes tend to reflect the IQ levels of their foster parents rather than those of their real parents. Evidence also exists that altering the diet of children may prohibit or reverse the behavior which is associated with mental retardation.[3]

Similarly, the physician's primary approach for treating hyperkinesis has been through the *p* factor, or the physiologic aspects of hyperkinesis, by changing the child's diet or through medication. The most obvious approach for the fields of psychology and education is through the *e*, or environmental aspects of hyperactivity, through different reading methods, structure, behavior modification, and dealing with the family constellation.

All of the above have dealt exclusively with one variable of the equation—either the *p* or the *e*. The eclectic approach we propose would encompass both, and thus open multiple options for the treatment of the behavior known as hyperkinesis. The physician would not be confined to the medication route, which often serves to keep him on the defensive. New possibilities would also be opened for educators, psychiatrists, and psychologists. These would allow for less manipulation of the child while at the same time place more focus on how certain behavior is created, magnified, and reinforced by the child's environment.

This eclectic approach would affect research as well as the treatment process. It proposes a more objective scrutinization of the problem, with more operationally defined terms. Rather than the broad, hazy entity labeled hyperkinesis, the narrow and singular aspects of the problem must be investigated. Specifically designated behavior should be measured under a variety of conditions. What must be avoided above all is a utilitarian approach, one creating a necessity to find research answers which comply with needed expectations.

We have taken a closer look at minimal brain dysfunction. We have suggested that the effectiveness of the agents used to control the behavior is very difficult to prove and that this is particularly true when we are dealing with behavior so poorly defined as hyperactivity and learning disability. Prudent researchers and statisticians are wary of the conclusions thus far derived. We suggest that both government and the drug industry be less willing to support individuals unqualified to do research in this field by reason of lack of appropriate training. Rather, support should be allocated to establish groups capable of carefully and deliberately planning and executing studies which can be replicated. In the meanwhile, those of us in the clinically applied field will be cautious in our conclusions and look more than ever before to alter the environment rather than the child.

References

1. Hewitt, F.: *The Emotionally Disturbed Child in the Classroom.* Allyn and Bacon, Boston, 1968, pp. 9–20.
2. Johnson, W.: The Indians Have No Word for It. *Q J Speech* **30:** 330–337, 1944.
3. Kirk, S.: *Educating Exceptional Children.* Houghton Mifflin, Boston, 1972, pp. 172–179.
4. Lewin, K.: *Principles of Topological Psychology.* McGraw-Hill, New York, 1936.
5. Marwit, S., and Stenner, A.: "Hyperkinesis: Delineation of Two Patterns," *Excep Child* **38:** 401–406, 1972.
6. Novack, H.: An Educator's View of Medication and Classroom Behavior. *J Learn Disabil* **4:** 43–45, 1971.
7. Rutter, M., et al.: *A Neuropsychiatric Study in Children.* J.B. Lippincott, Philadelphia, 1970, p. 190.
8. DeHirsch, K., et al.: *Predicting Reading Failure.* Harper & Row, New York, 1966, p. 85.

15

A Note of Caution Regarding the Use of Medication for School Problems

Lester Grinspoon, M.D.

At the very outset I should like to make clear that, the title of this chapter notwithstanding, I am not opposed to the use of amphetamines in the treatment of children suffering from hyperkinetic behavior disorders. My concern is with the inappropriate use of this drug in disturbed children. Second, there is the matter of bias—my bias. I approach the question of the utility of these drugs in the treatment of children with this disorder from the perspective of one who spent 3 years looking into every aspect of the amphetamines—the class of drug itself, its uses and abuses inside and outside of medicine, and its potential for harm. Over the course of this investigation, I have come to have less regard for its usefulness as a medicine and more respect for its capacity for harmfulness and abuse.

I hope that these two points will help to put into perspective my concern with the widespread use of amphetamines in the nation's schools to control the syndrome which doctors and medical researchers call *hyperkinetic behavior disorder* or *minimal brain dysfunction* and which teachers and parents know as *hyperactivity*. I have come

---

Associate Professor of Psychiatry, Harvard University Medical School, and Massachusetts Mental Health Center, Boston, Massachusetts.

to believe that enthusiasm in the administration of amphetamines has to some extent outstripped serious discussion about the efficacy of these drugs for treating children's behavioral disorders, and I fear that serious attempts to precisely define and diagnose the hyperkinetic impulse disorder have been supplanted by acceptance of drug therapy for large numbers of our school children, many of whom may not benefit from it. Amphetamines have become established as the preferred treatment in many school situations, even though doctors themselves remain unsure of the nature, etiology, and cure of hyperkinesis.

The attention of the public was brought to bear on the issue when, on June 29, 1970, a sensational article appeared in the *Washington Post* claiming that from 5 to 10 percent of the 62,000 grammar school children in Omaha, Nebraska, were being treated with "behavior modification drugs to improve classroom deportment and increase learning potential" (Omaha pupils given "behavior" drugs, 1970). Although the reported numbers were subsequently found to be greatly exaggerated—the 5 to 10 percent figure represented the estimated prevalence of learning disabilities among school children in Omaha[4] rather than the prevalence of amphetamine use—the article did excite public interest and concern about the increasingly widespread and largely unexamined practice of prescribing behavior control drugs. A number of hyperactive, easily distractible children in the Omaha school system were being treated with drugs, purportedly to help them learn better by slowing them down and allowing them to concentrate on their work. A rash of publicity following the appearance of the *Post* article disclosed that this practice was not limited to Nebraska, but was also taking place in a number of other states throughout the nation.

A Congressional hearing was convened on September 29, 1970, to investigate the extent of government involvement in this practice, and the testimonies of various respected government officials disclosed some disquieting facts. According to the testimony of Dr. Ronald Lipman of the Food and Drug Administration, some 150,000 to 200,000 children were then being treated with stimulant drugs and the trend was expected to increase in the future.[4] The National Institutes of Mental Health estimated that "there are up to 4 million 'hyperactive' children in the United States who could benefit from these drugs . . ."[7] Interest in the use of drugs for hyperactive children was gaining momentum despite the lack of follow-up studies on the long-term effects of the drugs. Until that time only one systematic follow-up study had been undertaken, directed by Connors and involving 67 children of 100 who at one time had been treated by Bradley, Denhoff, and Laufer. Preliminary results were reassuring; most of the children in the study who had been diagnosed as hyperkinetic and had received amphetamines showed a low incidence of psychiatric disorders in adolescence.[4,9] But Congressman Cornelius E. Gallagher, who chaired the hearing, was justifiably appalled that after 35 years of experience with drugs in the treatment of hyperkinesis, only one study involving 67 children could be produced to demonstrate the absence of harmful effects. Clearly this was too small a sample on which to base such a widespread practice.

Educators have become impressed with the possibilities offered by amphetamines and in many cases have been strong proponents of stimulant treatment for their problem students. In New York, the mother of a child labeled hyperactive by his elementary school teacher received an ultimatum from the teacher—"put the child on drugs or we will not be able to keep him in school."[5] A southern California mother reported her experience: "We've been harassed and pressured by the school for four years now to put our nine-year-old on medication—for hyperactivity—and we've refused for four years. Two family doctors have backed up our decision."[7] A Colorado mother told of how she had reluctantly "caved in to the combined requests of the school nurse, the school psychologist, principal, and teachers" to put her 6-year-old son on medication to treat his "learning disability." Another California mother complained that the school would not accept a "no" from the family physician. "Most every parent who has an overactive child in the school is told to go see the same pediatrician," she reported, "because that doctor knows what the school wants." Even in cases in which parents have not resisted and perhaps have even supported teachers' pressures to place their children on stimulants, a question still arises as to whether educators should have any authority to make such recommendations. In Baltimore, the use of amphetamines to treat unmanageable children in the city school system had reached such alarming proportions a few years ago that Dr. H. M. Selznick, then school system superintendent of special education, was forced to acknowledge that guidelines and controls about who should be responsible for the administration of the drugs were sorely lacking. And his apology continued, "We do not want teachers administering the drugs since they are not medically trained. But it is our opinion that some teachers who have had 'wall climbers' do assume this responsibility."[11]

Denhoff recognized this abuse as early as 1971. He wrote, "In the 1950s, educators learned about [the] . . . psychopharmacological aspects of behavior modification, and began to encourage parents to seek such help from the child's physician. Soon it became evident that these drugs were being used indiscriminately—prescription would depend mostly upon a description of behavior by a teacher or parent."[1]

With politically inspired, emotionally charged publicity surrounding and following the Gallagher hearings, the public was alerted to the extensive abuse without being given any solid scientific facts to temper their reaction. Yet the transcript of the hearings demonstrates that such reassuring facts were generally not available even from those government officials whose job it is to regulate the use of drugs. Instead it became clear that amphetamines have been abused in the name of therapy for children. While psychiatrists' estimates of the prevalence of hyperkinesis among elementary school children range from 4 to 10% at a maximum,[3,6,15,16,17] educators estimate the incidence to be as high as 15–20%.

Not much has changed. The issues remain emotionally charged, and information is still lacking about the hyperkinetic state as it is diagnosed technically by medical doctors and as it is identified in the schools. The need for clear policy recommendations persists. How should parents, teachers, doctors, and concerned policy-makers respond? What steps can citizens take beyond mere acceptance or indignation? What might be an enlightened policy regarding treatment of hyperkinesis? There is no question that a serious reevaluation of current practices is needed before society proceeds in dispensing psychoactive drugs to its children.

A major concern is that the use of drugs to "modify" classroom behavior constitutes a covert subversion of what our educational ideals *should* be. If an important aim of our educational institutions were really to help young people deal with and learn to regulate their "self-destructive" or even "antisocial" tendencies, it would make little sense to give them drugs as soon as they exhibited restless or unruly behavior. Students and, perhaps especially, those at the elementary level need and deserve educational environments designed to help them come to grips with their natural dispositions and learn to use in a certain way what Phillip Jackson at the University of Chicago has nicely called their own executive powers: "Any form of intervention that relieves the restless or unruly child of the need, or deprives him of the opportunity, to use his executive powers deprives him to that extent of the chance to develop insight and skill in self-control."[8]

There is no doubt that the behavior taken as a sign of hyperkinesis is real enough. Restless, angry, disturbed, and inattentive students constitute a major problem for many parents and teachers. It also may be true that some elementary school children exhibit this kind of behavior because of organic brain damage or neurohormonal insufficiencies. But it is impossible to believe that the hundreds of thousands of school children who are now being routinely administered stimulants are *all* suffering from organic brain damage or deficiencies in crucial CNS neurohormones. There is no justification for the increasingly popular leap from the observation of disruptive or inattentive behavior to the supposition that this is the result of a specific disorder of the central nervous system. Nor does the observation that amphetamines sometimes reduce disruptiveness and increase attention provide any grounds for supposing that even these are true cases of organically based hyperkinesis. Amphetamines can affect behavior and learning problems of psychogenic and environmental etiology in much the same way as they affect problems presumed to have an organic basis.

Our society has been undergoing a critical upheaval in values. Children growing up in the past decade have seen claims to authority and existing institutions questioned as an everyday occurrence, and the classroom has become a major stage on which this value upheaval is played out. Teachers no longer have the unquestioned authority they once had in the classroom, nor do they have at their disposal many well-defined ways of relating to children not based on their presumed authority. The child, on the other side, is no longer so intimidated by whatever authority the teacher has, and demands, often through his behavior, to be acknowledged as an individual and treated with concern. Hyperkinesis, whatever organic condition it may legitimately refer to, has become a convenient label with which to dismiss this phenomenon as a physical disease rather than treating it as the social problem it is. The use of drugs, particularly amphetamines, in the name of therapy, often does little more than provide a relatively easy and economical way of making the classroom situation more tolerable and manageable for the teacher.

We should also be concerned about how much attention is being paid to possible alternatives to drug therapy which may be both safer and more effective in the long run. For example, in 1971 Alvin Toffler reported to the American Psychological Association on the results of a series of experiments using easily learned classroom behavior modification techniques on groups of hyperactive children with either normal or abnormal EEG tracings.[12] After 24 hyperactive elementary school children with normal IQs had been administered complete EEGs they were given simple reinforcement for attentiveness to an academic workbook task in an experimental classroom environment. Their rates of attentiveness, cooperation, and accuracy were measured before, during, and after the application of simple positive reinforcement techniques of praise and reward. These disturbed children consistently showed significant decreases in hyperactivity after behavior modification therapy and the improvement carried over into their regular school environments. One of the more interesting findings was that the students with abnormal EEGs showed considerable and highly significant decreases in hyperactivity and increases in overall classroom performance as compared with the students who had been judged hyperactive but had normal EEGs, even though the latter students also showed marked improvement. No such improvement was noted in a non-treated control group of similarly "disturbed" or hyperactive children (with or without normal EEGs). Toffler concluded that before initiating amphetamine or other drug therapy and before attempting any depth psychotherapy or even "special class" placement, simple behavior modification techniques should be attempted for even the most severely agitated hyperkinetics, since it is their *behavior* which is almost always the criterion by which they are judged psychologically or organically "sick," "deviant," or "deficient." Werry and Sprague support this conclusion in their recommendation that drugs ". . . should not be used as the only or even the primary treatment, except where circumstances preclude behavior modification techniques."[19] Behavior modification techniques, while they are no panacea and have their own significant potential for abuse, do have this virtue: their proper application requires on the part of those who employ them a sensitivity to the needs, talents, and preferences of the individual child. Rather than simply making children more manageable, as drugs often do, such techniques may bring out their best qualities. Moreover, these techniques allow the children to discover their impulses and to make use of their own powers of self-control in dealing with them. They do not just abolish temporarily the more disturbing impulses, thereby rendering control unnecessary. Behavior learned through the use of such techniques potentially can be generalized to many situations beyond the specific situation in which the behavior was originally conditioned.[2,14] In contrast, drug-facilitated learning not only is not generalized to a broad spectrum of situations but evidence suggests that it is actually forgotten quite readily.[10,13,18]

None of this is to deny the possibility that there is a true, organically based hyperkinesis which may benefit from drug treatment. It is time, however, that we take an honest look at the evidence to date and admit that where such a disorder exists it is difficult to distinguish it from other syndromes or disturbances which are expressed by similar behavioral patterns. Symptoms, not causes, have become the focus of treatment, creating a significant potential for abuse.

References

1. Denhoff, E.: To medicate—to debate—or to validate. *J Learn Disabil* **4:** 467–469, 1971.
2. Doubros, S.G., and Daniels, G.J.: An experimental approach to the reduction of overactive behavior. *Behav Res Ther* **4:** 251–258, 1966.
3. Eisenberg, L.: The hyperkinetic child and stimulant drugs. *N Engl J Med* **287:** 249–250, 1972.
4. Federal involvement in the use of behavior modification drugs on grammar school children of the right to privacy inquiry. Hearing before a subcommittee of the Committee on Government Operations, House of Representatives, 91st Congress, 2nd Session, September 29, 1970. U.S. Government Printing Office, Washington, D.C., 1970.
5. Hentoff, N.: Drug-pushing in the schools: The professionals (I). *Village Voice*, May 25, 1972, pp. 20–22.
6. Huessey, H.R.: Study of the prevalence and therapy of the hyperkinetic syndrome in public school children in rural Vermont. *Acta Paedopsychiatr* **34:** 130–135, 1967.
7. Hunsinger, S.: School storm: Drugs for children. *Christian Science Monitor*, October 31, 1970, pp, 1, 6.
8. Ladd, E.T.: Pills for classroom peace. *Saturday Review*, November 21, 1970, pp. 66–68, 81–83.
9. Laufer, M.W.: Long-term management and some follow-up findings on the use of drugs with minimal cerebral syndromes. *J Learn Disabil* **4:** 518–522, 1971.
10. Miller, N.E.: Some animal experiments pertinent to the problem of combining psychotherapy with drug therapy. *Compr Psychiatry* **7:** 1–12, 1966.
11. Miller, S.: Use of tranquilizers by city pupils reported increasing. *Baltimore Evening Sun*, October 2, 1970.
12. Novack, H.S.: An educator's view of medication and classroom behavior. *J Learn Disabil* **4:** 507–508, 1971.
13. Overton, D.A.: State-dependent learning produced by depressant and atropine-like drugs. *Psychopharmacologia (Berlin)* **10:** 6–31, 1966.
14. Patterson, G.R., Jones, R., Whittier, J., and Wright, M.A.: A behavior modification technique for the hyperactive child. *Behav Res Ther* **2:** 217–226, 1965.
15. Prechtl, H.F.R., and Stemmer, C.J.: The choreiform syndrome in children. *Dev Med Child Neurol* **4:** 119–127, 1962.
16. Stewart, M.A.: Hyperactive children. *Sci Am* **222:** 94–98, 1970.
17. Stewart, M.A., Pitts, F.N., Craig, A.G., and Dierof, N.: The hyperactive child syndrome. *Am J Orthopsychiatry* **36:** 861–867, 1966.
18. Turner, R.K.: CNS stimulant drugs and conditioning treatment of nocturnal enuresis: A long-term follow-up study. *Behav Res Ther* **4:** 225–228, 1966.
19. Werry, J.S., and Sprague, R.L.: Hyperactivity. In *Symptoms of psychopathology*, C.G. Costello, Ed., Wiley, New York, 1970, p. 408.

16

Minimal Brain Dysfunction: Ethical Issues, Treatment, and Medical Evidence

Robert E. Cooke, M.D.

I would prefer to discuss rather than deliver a sermon on this problem because I think the issues are very much ones which have no clear-cut answers. I have attempted to reconcile the differences between the participants. I recognize the problems of the affected child and the hardships for him and his family. I recognize the inappropriate and inadequate management in school, which certainly exists in many situations. I agree, but also disagree in part, with the view that there are indeed some serious abuses of public action. When one abandons science and becomes an ethicist, an amateur one as I have become, the easiest thing is to say nothing. If you were to ask me whether drugs are a good idea or not, I would reply, "Yes or no, but don't quote me."

Drugs in the treatment of the hyperactive child present ethical dilemmas which have already been pointed out very effectively. They are not, however, unique to minimal brain dysfunction. One sees these same kinds of problems in other types of patients with various emotional problems. Critics describe drugs as destroying will power. Another view holds that they should be an adjunctive accessory. On

---

President, Medical College of Pennsylvania, Philadelphia, Pennsylvania.

the other hand, Dr. Kinsbourne has said that they normalize behavior. Enthusiasts say they liberate potential enslaved by illness. Court actions have forced the right to treatment of the mentally handicapped, and at the same time have upheld the right of parents and guardians as well as the patients themselves to refuse treatment. Those who have dealt with a chronic schizophrenic will realize that they are probably in the most need of new experimental therapeutic approaches, yet they may be very handicapped in giving consistent informed consent. Obviously there are serious dilemmas in this area.

In regard to psychostimulants questions are raised, such as: are these drugs a cheap and dehumanizing way of minimizing problems caused by poor schooling, poor parenting, and poor environment? Are drugs a substitute for social and educational interventions that are expensive and difficult to initiate?

Are creative and original future leaders, "possibly latent geniuses" to quote one author, being suppressed by our flagrant use of drugs as therapy? Should 90 percent of children in certain slum areas of Baltimore be candidates for stimulant drug therapy, as Paul Wender has suggested they might be? The answers to such questions require serious ethical reflection as opposed to a cavalier approach.

In this regard, what helps the greatest number is not necessarily the best treatment. Whatever does the most good for the greatest number is possibly, and *I want to emphasize this, possibly*, but not necessarily, right. It certainly would be right if utility were our only principle, if all that mattered were consequences. However, I do not believe that is the only principle we abide by in medicine. Other ethical principles are just as important. Surely, every effort must be made to do good. That is beneficience and true utility. But every effort must also be made to minimize harm, the principle of non-injury. Every effort must also be made to be fair and just, and to respect the individual and respect his autonomy. Every effort should be made to tell the truth because this is the basis of trust.

Using such principles, let us look at the medical issues that relate to the administration of stimulant drugs to the hyperactive child. I think these issues are best illustrated by a series of questions.

First, Is the use of Ritalin or Dexedrine in minimal brain dysfunction a valid practice? Is the evidence sufficient to warrant their use in at least some particular types of patients? I think the evidence so far would probably indicate "yes." If carefully controlled studies show clearly and without doubt the benefit and the lack of harm in certain types of patients, I think the answer is clearly yes, at least in the short run, in certain types of patients. Some children change their behavior dramatically under the influence of stimulant drugs, and some of the tests of Kinsbourne and his colleagues are objective evidence of this. They do this far more frequently than with placebos and with relatively little short-term toxicity. Unfortunately, in the long term the data as regards benefit or harm are not as adequate.

This is not surprising: Eugene Stedd, a great figure in American medicine, pointed out that the most difficult problem in research is treatment of chronic disorders because of the enormous number of variables that occur over time. If we make the assumption that the use of stimulant drugs is effective in certain children and in that sense is a valid practice in those children, what is necessary to prevent misuse?

I suggest four steps that we must follow if we are to ensure appropriate usage.

1. It is essential to avoid a vague diagnosis. We must utilize as much as possible the criteria that can identify the child as belonging to the group that has been benefited. Careful evaluation and diagnosis of the child, the school, and the family is absolutely essential; the drug should not be administered as a therapeutic test. The idea that a successful trial of the drug proves the diagnosis is unacceptable. A careful look for the excessive activity, and an evaluation of the serious attention problems, the perceptual/motor difficulty, the impulsiveness, the clumsiness, etc., so beautifully described by the parents earlier in this book, are necessary ingredients for validating the use of medication.

2. It is essential to determine if the problem is serious enough to warrant therapy. Is there enough discomfort to the child, who bears the risk, and not just to the anxious parents or harassed teachers? Is the child so inattentive despite the use of other less risky measures that he is seriously handicapped?

3. The therapy must be for the benefit of the child. Is is a substitute for a sedative for the teacher, psychotherapy for the mother, or family counseling for the father? The primary principle underlying the care of all children is to do good and to minimize harm. I also like to visualize as a consequence of being fair and being just, as a derivative of distributive justice, an obligation on the part of adults in society to help children. This should be more than just a legal or moral right of children since there seems to be no end to the number of rights claimed by our society: the right to work, the right to health, the right to treatment, the right to happiness, the right to play golf on Sunday, etc. Parents and teachers, in theory at least, have an obligation to tolerate all forms of behavior in their children, but they, like all of us, may have a limited capacity to fulfill that obligation. Indeed, in the case of the truly hyperactive child, and I certainly

think that the patient described here is an example, few parents or few teachers have such a capacity. The distinction as to who benefits most is not easy to make. Overactivity produces low attentiveness, with school failure. Reduced motivation results in parental conflicts. Improvement alters the regard of others which in turn improves self-regard, particularly in the child with low self-esteem. More success prompts greater exploration and improved motivation and more acceptance by others. Who benefits most—the child, the parents, or the teacher—may not be easy to determine.

4. If it is essential that the decision to treat not be made lightly, who then should make the decision? In the early years of their child's life, parents clearly make almost all behavior-controlling decisions, acting in theory in the best interests of the child, by using reward and punishment and by setting an example. Society does not get involved unless there is serious physical harm, as in the case of child abuse, which is the best example of societal intervention.

In the mid-years of childhood, teachers make most of the behavior-controlling decisions, acting in theory in the best interest of the child and society, again by using rewards, punishment, and example. This persists until the adolescent period, when to a large extent peers take over from both the parents and teachers. In this regard the question must be asked whether behavior-controlling decisions by parents or teachers extend to the use of stimulant or other psychoactive drugs. If a parent or teacher wishes a child to have stimulant drugs, is the physician or pharmacist obligated to supply them? My answer is no, quite clearly. These are not over-the-counter drugs in that technical sense, and for good reason. They are not to be used indiscriminately. Careful diagnosis is necessary, even though it may be imperfect and difficult. Monitoring for harmful side effects is necessary. Parents cannot and teachers should not be solely responsible for decision-making when it comes to prescribing medication. However, they should be involved in the decision to administer or withhold stimulant drugs, although some conflict of interest does exist. Thus, although there is a large professional and scientific component to be considered, there are enough social and moral implications to warrant careful consideration by all involved in the caretaking process. In such circumstances, I find it useful to consider how the ideal judge makes decisions under Roderick Firth's ideal observer theory. The ideal judge is one who is omniscient and omnipercipient, that is, he perceives how all others are affected by the decision. He is dispassionate and disinterested. Obviously, even our best legal minds do not fit that description, but omniscience can be approximated to an extent by the professional presenting scientific data. The parents, teachers, social workers, and the nurse all may be able to assist in determining how others are affected by this behavior and by change. Group participation tends to cancel out biases, and this allows impartiality. I think that such team decision-making is not uncommon in treatment of the learning-disabled child. The social worker, the nurse, the teacher, the parent, the psychologist, the psychiatrist, the neurologist, and the pediatrician together can possibly work out a plan that meets most of the principles for the ideal judge I have described. The physician is finally legally responsible for prescribing drugs and makes the final determination, but it is hoped that he or she uses group decision models in which all options, not simply drug therapy, are considered.

Unfortunately, or possibly fortunately for some, the dilemma does not stop at that point. What if there are theoretically better approaches to the problem? Should society, the physicians, the psychopharmacologist, the psychologist, or the educator stop using existing methods of treatment? Are there better drugs? Are there better ways to treat than with the use of drugs? Benjamin Feingold has asked an interesting question: What do food additives do? Does behavior modification with drug therapy make a substantial difference, or just behavior modification alone? Such questions will continue to arise. To minimize harm, to maximize benefit, to be just in offering benefits from science, and to respect the individual, other interventions must be explored. Yet people have a wide range of attitudes regarding human experience and human experimentation in general and drug testing in particular. I think the question is best put as: is there a moral obligation for research? Paul Ramsey, a conservative, says no and has an interesting approach. He says, "Our descendents do not have a right, namely a moral claim to new miracle cures. We will not have sinned against them (our descendents) if arthritis is not cured." Dyke and Richardson at the Harvard Divinity School look at it differently. They say that using human subjects in research with some risk is not only morally justified but in certain instances is morally required. The moral grounds are the limitation of animal research and the stringent moral demands to alleviate suffering. There is an important caveat, however, and this is frequently ignored. Benefits must not be luxury items but must save life or reduce the threat of death, much suffering, much discomfort, or serious unhappiness rather than just give greater pleasure. Under the rubric of greater pleasure one can justify almost anything.

What ethical issues then arise in carrying out such research? If a diet without food additives is to be tested, is it justified to withdraw drug therapy when it seems to be effective? Is it justified, even though necessary to provide clear-cut answers to the question of benefit from special diets, to have a control group off drugs and receiving food additives? Is it ethical to stop supposedly effective treatment in this condition and substitute some other that may or may not be helpful? Can parents consent on behalf of the child to stop therapy when the substitute may be less effective? Apomorphine has been mentioned as a possible therapeutic approach. How can this be studied? Can parents ethically consent to such a new research approach involving a drug? We have heard that parents evidently ethically consented for normal children to receive stimulants as part of Dr. Kinsbourne's study. However, only by such controlled studies can useless or even harmful interventions be kept from being accepted, though unvalidated, practices. It is certainly correct that there may be unvalidated practices which have become widely accepted.

Controlled studies contain their own ethical dilemmas, however. In testing a substitute for stimulants that may be less toxic by studies in animals or adults, who can consent for children? Is the placebo trial indicated? Answers to such questions come from the application of the same ethical principles as apply to practice—doing good, minimizing harm, being fair, and being truthful. If there is substantial reason to believe that more benefit will accrue to the subject from the use of one approach than the use of another, then is it justified to compare these? Some benefits, for example, may come from placebos and yet there is no risk. On the other hand, there may be risk with drugs and no benefit. There should be no discrimination in the selection of subjects. The child in an institution who is more readily studied because the parents will not object is not fair game for research. The risk as well as the benefits must be widely distributed. If a control subject is given a placebo and there is benefit to the treated group, then a crossover must be carried out from the placebo group to the treated group to ensure fairness in the offering of opportunities for participation. That term is used instead of the usual "recruitment of subjects." Truth telling is essential in research as well as in practice. Parents must know that their children may receive an active or less active agent and how the selection will be made. The potential risks and benefits as well as the probabilities should be thoroughly explained. If an investigator firmly believes that one group or another in the research design clearly stands to benefit far more than the other, then the study is unethical and should not be conducted. If the investigator can honestly say, "I do not know which group I would wish to be enrolled in," then the study is justified. All must be aware of the possibilities, and the agreement of the subject should be sought if he or she is old enough to understand some of the aspects of treatment. If the intent is to benefit the subject, and the risk of harm is low, parents may give substituted judgment, just as they do in so many more hazardous activities on behalf of their child; if there is no intention of benefiting the child such as in phase 1 drug trials, then substituted consent is not in order if there is any significant risk.

Finally we come to the translation of research into practice. When is research on treatment convincing enough to validate that treatment? One of our problems now is that there are no general rules. When I was a house officer at Yale in 1944 I was the first to treat a case of tuberculous meningitis with streptomycin. That one case validated the therapy because the diagnosis was clear-cut, the disease had been 100 percent fatal, the bacilli disappeared rapidly, and animal studies had indicated the effectiveness of streptomycin against tuberculosis. Streptomycin became validated therapy instantly. But with minimal brain dysfunction the situation is far more difficult. The manifestations are more variable and the symptoms are heavily socially dependent and may even be more severe or at times absent in a different environment, at least for a brief while. Several therapeutic approaches are possible; even placebos are effective in a fairly high percentage of subjects. How many studies with what numbers of subjects using what statistical methods and what objective criteria are necessary to convince the majority of practitioners and the public? Obviously no hard and fast answers can be given in this instance or in many others.

Hopefully, in the case of the hyperactive children and those with minimal brain dysfunction syndrome, carefully controlled research, with adequate numbers over long periods will be performed to clarify what continues as a practical dilemma. Such studies would seem to me to be a highly valuable product of this symposium. Carrying them out would not be easy, but the benefits to many children everywhere would be considerable. With the extent of controversy that exists, federal support would seem to be almost obligatory. Only when the results of such long-term study are common knowledge will the many complaints be stilled.

Summary and Conclusions

There is increasing concern in society that subjects, particularly children, are being exploited; yet, at the same time there is concern that the benefits to biomedical science are not being brought rapidly enough to the public.

Are drugs a cheap and dehumanizing way of minimizing problems caused by poor schooling, poor parenting, and poor environments?

Or, do drugs normalize behavior and liberate the potential enslaved by illness? The answers to such questions require serious ethical reflection, and good ethics always begins with good data.

In regard to the use of psychostimulants such as methylphenidate, carefully controlled studies have shown substantial benefit and lack of harm in certain types of patients for periods of weeks or months. Certain children demonstrate marked changes in behavior under the influence of stimulant drugs far more frequently than with placebos. In the use of such drugs it is essential to avoid inaccurate diagnosis; they must be used only in serious, not trivial, problems; the therapy must be for the benefit of the child not his caretakers; and the decision must not be made lightly.

Such requirements imply that the physician, only after full consultation with teachers, parents, social workers, psychologists, and others, embarks on a therapeutic trial. Team evaluation for the child with minimal brain dysfunction becomes a necessity not a luxury and the cavalier administration of such drugs by educators or health professionals must be discontinued. Further research on the long-term benefits and potential for harm must be encouraged.

Name Index

Institution Index

Subject Index